Bethesda G

How to be a Truly EXCELLENT Junior Medical Student

7th edition

Robert J. Lederman, MD

TABLE OF CONTENTS

Introduction	1
How a Hospital Works	2
Outpatient versus Inpatient Care	2
Community versus Teaching Hospitals	2
Private and Staff Patients	3
Nursing Units and Specialty Services	4
Nursing Unit Personnel	4
Physician Teams	8
Getting Admitted to the Hospital	11
Night Call	13
Ward Routines from a Patient's Perspective	14
How to DO stuff	18
The Chart Review	18

How to be a Truly Excellent Junior Medical Student

Orders	21
Medications & Prescriptions	37
Wash your hands and instruments	47
Writing Notes	48
Admission Notes	48
Copying-forward notes in electronic health records	53
Internal Medicine Daily Progress Notes	55
Discharge Notes	58
Surgery	59
Obstetrics	67
Pediatrics	71
Neurology	74
Psychiatry	78
Procedures	81
Preparing for any procedure	81
Introduction to Phlebotomy & IV Placement	84
Performing venipuncture	89
Placing IV's	92
Blood Culture	98
Arterial Blood Gas	100
Electrocardiograms	104
Lumbar Puncture	105
Nasogastric Tube (NG) and Dobhoff placement	106
Placing a Urinary (Foley) Catheter	110
Procedure Notes	113
Local Anesthesia	114
Imaging Tests	115
Bedside Tests	116
Urinalysis	116
Gram Stain	123
How to be organized and compulsive	127
Organizing your data and your schedule	127
Presentations	130
Index	139

How to be a Truly Excellent Junior Medical Student

Disclaimer I mean this book to be truthful and useful. You are responsible for any decisions you make or actions you take, irrespective of what this book says. Moreover, the distributor of this book has reserved the right to modify it without notice to the author or reader. This is the world we live in. Therefore, we must disclaim liability for loss or damage caused by your using this book.

If you do not accept this disclaimer, please return the book immediately for a refund.

Robert J. Lederman, MD, Cardiovascular Branch, Division of Intramural Research, National Heart Lung and Blood Institute, National Institutes of Health, Bethesda, Maryland USA. E-mail: robert.lederman@gmail.com.

This book was authored by Robert J. Lederman in his private capacity. The views expressed in this book are the author's own, and do not necessarily represent the views of NIH, DHHS, nor the United States.

How to be a Truly EXCELLENT Junior Medical Student
ISBN 9781686997921. Copyright © 2019 Robert J. Lederman, MD. All rights reserved. Printed in the USA. Published by Bethesda Guides, Bethesda, Maryland, USA.

Preface to the 7th Edition

This book has remained a hit even though it has been two decades since the last edition. Medicine has evolved in the interim with the introduction of electronic health records and order entry, restrictions on "non-accredited" bedside laboratory testing, and trainee work hour restrictions.

In the 7th edition I have decided to retain much of the old-fashioned techniques (data entry, procedure methods, and bedside testing methods) to give new medical students a flavor of what goes into the making of "the sausage" that is contemporary medical care.

Dedications

To my son Adam and my wife Laura.

Blessings to Beth O'Toole and Beth Benson for guiding me on the wards when I was a medical student, and to Lee Biblo and Keith Armitage thereafter.

Thanks to Patrick Javid and Jennifer Zelenock for their contributions a few years back.

This book is dedicated to my brother Michael Lederman who showed me what it means to be a physician.

Cover Images

The Anatomy Lesson of Dr. Nicolaes Tulp. Oil on canvas, 2013, by Rembrandt. Mauritshuis museum in The Hague, Netherlands

Introduction

Ward medicine may easily intimidate you when you begin your third year of medical school. Medical and social disasters abound; many require decisive action. Your teachers — attendings and residents — are often distracted. Nurses, paraprofessionals, and even patients may ignore you. The hours are probably much longer than you are accustomed to. Although you have been studying medicine for years, you may arrive with few skills immediately useful to the health care team.

It is not surprising that most new **Junior Medical Students** (JMS) are entirely unlike themselves during their first few clerkships. Fear is in their eyes. Their movements are awkward. Their interactions with patients are stiff. They've lost the common sense and gracefulness they had beforehand.

This guide was written in an attempt to make **your** first few months of clinical clerkships less disorienting and frightening. The sooner you feel at ease, the sooner your common sense will return and the sooner you will function effectively on the wards.

Do not be frightened by the details! You are not expected to begin your clerkships already knowing this sort of material.

How to be a truly EXCELLENT Junior Medical Student is an introduction to clinical clerkships, not a textbook of patient care. While I have attempted to provide accurate and up-to-date information, you should never substitute this guide for your supervisors' guidance.

A note on work hour restrictions

It does not take long to realize that any patient would prefer the care of a fatigued but wizened trainee over a well-rested dolt. In a well-intentioned response to intuition and poorly designed experiments, medical students are often denied the opportunity to spend "enough" time with patients and staff to garner experience. My strong advice to you is to find a way to surmount this onerous challenge: go home and study. Think about your patients and their problems. Plan your next moves so that every moment on the wards is well-spent.

How a Hospital Works
Outpatient versus Inpatient Care

You will spend the bulk of your student clerkships at inpatient facilities (hospitals). However, most health care in this country happens at outpatient facilities: doctors' offices, clinics, and emergency departments. Training in a hospital skews your experience towards acute and serious illness.

Your encounters with hospital patients represent only a small part of their health care, which may consist of any combination of outpatient, inpatient, and assisted care (*e.g.,* home health care or nursing homes).

In addition to inpatient beds, most hospitals have outpatient facilities. Outpatient facilities may include an emergency department, private physicians' offices, clinics for routine ambulatory, and specialty clinics for patients with a defined spectrum of problems, such as a neurology clinic or a diabetes clinic.

Keep in mind that before admission, all hospital patients were screened at an outpatient facility or emergency department. A report from this screening is an important source of historical information about your patient.

Community versus Teaching Hospitals

In most community hospitals patients are under the direct care of private physicians. In these hospitals, physicians admit their own patients, visit them regularly, and leave instructions for care with the nursing staff. When problems arise, nurses call these physicians for advice and new instructions.

Teaching hospitals, like the ones that train Junior Medical Students, work very differently. Patients in these hospitals are under the direct care of physicians-in-training, **house officers**. These include **interns**, who are first-year MD's, and **residents**, who have completed internship.

Interns evaluate patients admitted to their teams and act as the primary physician for these patients. Interns rely on residents for advice and supervision. Residents usually oversee several interns and junior residents, acting as the team leader and liaison to the attending physician.

Senior physicians, known as attendings, supervise entire teams of house officers. These ward attendings guide house officer decision-making by intervening when they anticipate mistakes. Their primary role is educational. Most attendings are salaried faculty members, although some are part-time faculty who spend the rest of their time managing private practices. It can get confusing, because some full-time faculty attendings also have private practices.

Other attendings do not supervise ward teams. These attendings are private physicians who have admitting privileges to the teaching hospital. House officers care for these private patients in return for guidance and teaching.

It is important to remember that attending physicians are ultimately responsible for all medical care under their supervision; their decisions prevail.

Private and Staff Patients

Most teaching hospitals have two categories of patients: private and staff.

Private patients often have long-standing relationships with private attendings or have been referred for care by specific private attendings. Private attendings direct major decisions, but house officers evaluate the patients independently and tend to hour-by-hour problems. House officers *must* confer with the attending whenever important therapeutic or procedural decisions are made.

Staff patients have no personal physicians or come to the hospital without referral from one. House officers assume a greater responsibility for their care, and play a greater role in important decisions. The attending-on-service is ultimately responsible for staff patients but for the sake of training may give house officers considerable latitude in decision-making. At some institutions, interns serve as personal doctors for staff patients and continue to follow them in outpatient clinics after discharge. At some institutions, for example, at Veterans Administration hospitals, all patients are considered staff patients. As a JMS you may interact more with your attending if you follow staff patients, since ward attendings pay particular attention to these patients.

> Follow staff patients whenever possible.

Nursing Units and Specialty Services

When patients are admitted for inpatient care, they are sent to nursing units according to the type and level of care they need. The units are organized around the manpower and skills of the nursing staff, which allow patients to be put under the care of discrete teams of physicians, nurses, and paraprofessionals. Patients are sent to nursing units according to the type and level of care they need. For example, patients with obstetrical problems are sent to obstetrical units, where nurses and doctors have experience with obstetrical care. Patients with critical medical problems are sent to medical intensive care units where highly experienced and specially trained nurses provide very close attention. Those with less critical medical problems are sent to medical wards, where individual nurses care for a larger number of patients.

Most large hospitals have nursing units for each medical specialty: surgery, obstetrics & gynecology, internal medicine, pediatrics, and psychiatry. Most also have intensive care units and some have subspecialty services, like oncology units, cardiac care units, geriatric units, *etc*.

Nursing Unit Personnel

The nursing unit is staffed by three teams, each with different responsibilities for patient care:

- Physicians, including attendings, fellows, house officers, and students.
- New to these teams are positions such as registered nurse practitioners and physician assistants (PA's) who may function much like residents.
- Nurses, nursing technicians, nursing students, and therapists.

- "Ancillary" staff, including secretaries, technicians, transporters, custodians.

House officers and attendings direct patient care but may deliver surprisingly little of it personally. Nurses and ancillary staff have the most contact with patients. If you do not work well with them, both you and your patients will be miserable.

Ward Secretary

The ward secretary "runs the show" in the nursing unit by managing the day-to-day administrative operation.

Depending on the institution, the ward secretary welcomes family visitors, coordinates communications during patient emergencies, contacts messengers to transport patients or specimens, summons technicians, schedules post-discharge appointments, notifies nurses and house officers of impending admissions, orders patient meals, answers intercoms from patients, answers the telephone, manages supplies, and much more.

Ward secretaries have the uncanny ability to process medical information without any medical training, to hold several simultaneous conversations, and to hear you without giving any hint of paying attention to you.

When house officers and medical students do not get along with the ward secretary, things do not operate smoothly. Always promote good will with the ward secretary.

Nurses

> Pay attention to nurses.
>
> Read nursing notes.
>
> Take heed when a nurse is apprehensive about a patient; something important is probably wrong.

Nurses are patients' primary caregivers. They must carry out physician orders or account for discrepancies. Nurses administer drugs, IV fluids, and parenteral nutrition. With the help of nursing technicians, nurses care for wounds and catheters, obtain specimens, bathe and toilet patients, and collect vital signs and other clinical measurements, *etc.* Nurses teach patients and families about disease and care, and they soothe their apprehensions. Of all the ward staff, nurses spend the most time talking to patients and tending to their needs. Not surprisingly, they are often the first to spot a deterioration in the patient's condition.

Many medical students do not realize how difficult nursing is, how hard nurses work, or how valuable their input is in patient care. Too many students and doctors are disrespectful to nurses, interfering with their patient relationships, adding unnecessarily to their workload, and ignoring their recommendations. Avoid these mistakes.

Respiratory Therapists
Respiratory therapists adjust mechanical ventilator settings in ICU patients, maintain oxygen delivery systems, administer nebulized drug therapy (*e.g.,* bronchodilators or antimicrobials), perform postural drainage and clapping maneuvers for pulmonary toilet, run pulmonary function and arterial blood gas (ABG) laboratories, sometimes obtain ABG specimens, and obtain pulse-oximeter measurements.

Technicians: IV, Phlebotomy, ECG, Portable tests
Some hospitals have technicians available to perform tests quickly and reproducibly. You should learn to do most of these things yourself, since technicians often are not available during wee hours, in emergencies, or at VA or county hospitals. Get to know the technicians. They can teach you many tricks. They can also help you get things done more quickly and smoothly for your patients.

Dietitians
Dietitians review the nutrition and intake of patients. They recommend regimens for patients with specific dietary restrictions, like patients with renal failure or diabetes. They are very knowledgeable about parenteral alimentation (IV feedings) and about forced enteral (nasogastric) feeding. You can ask the nutrition staff to count the calories your patients are consuming when you are unsure how much they are really eating. As you will see, dietary

management can get very tricky. Dietitians are an underutilized resource. Take advantage of their services.

Pharmacists

Pharmacists usually know much more about drug therapy than do house officers. At many hospitals, nursing units employ full-time doctors of pharmacology (Pharm.D.) who round with the physician teams. Pharm.D's make sure dangerous or expensive drugs are used properly. Call upon them when you have questions about drug dosages, drug interactions, or other recommended therapies.

Physical and Occupational Therapists

Physical therapists work with patients to maintain mobility and strength. They help patients exercise limbs after orthopedic surgery, mobilize joints when at risk of contracture, exercise when otherwise bedridden, and walk when recovering from stroke or when using a walker, cane, or crutch.

Occupational therapists help patients who are physically impaired function more independently. Occupational therapists concentrate on activities of daily living and on fine motor skills. For example, they may help a stroke patient re-learn how to bathe, dress, or hold a spoon.

Social Workers

Social workers are troubleshooters for patients' non-medical problems. They make sure families are equipped to care for patients after discharge. They arrange home health care visits by nurses or nursing aides. They arrange placement in nursing homes and rehabilitation centers. They help indigent and elderly patients apply for government health assistance and supplemental income programs. Social workers may intervene in difficult family situations, especially on pediatric units. On psychiatric units, social workers assume an especially active role in routine patient evaluation and management.

Good social workers dramatically lighten the workload of the rest of the medical team. Often the problems social workers solve are the same problems that keep a patient in the hospital long after they are medically ready to leave.

Advanced Practice Providers, aka Physician Assistants (PA's) and Nurse Practitioners (NP's)

These health care providers are seen in both outpatient clinics and inpatient wards. PA's and NP's often see their own patients, make diagnostic recommendations, and prescribe medication under the supervision of physicians. In addition, PA's and NP's play an integral role on inpatient medical teams, assisting with patient histories, physical exams, progress notes, and discharge planning. Think of them as full-time residents.

Physician Teams

Physician teams consist of interns and medical students led by residents, all supervised by attendings.

Interns

Internship is considered the most difficult year of medical training. Interns have an especially tough time early in the academic year: they may be new to the institution, unfamiliar with hospital routines and personalities, unprepared for the workload and sleep deprivation, new to the city, and lonely. Having little practical experience, they suddenly become the primary physicians for a large number of patients.

Interns work very hard to take good care of their patients. However, you should understand some of their more mundane priorities if you want to get along well with them:

- To finish daily care of patients as quickly as possible.
- To evaluate and initiate therapy for each new patient.
- To discharge or transfer patients from their care as soon as possible, thereby reducing the number of patients for whom they are responsible.
- To minimize unimportant calls and distractions from nurses.
- To insure smooth flow of ward activities.
- To sleep.

Some interns view any distraction from these goals either as an annoyance or as charity.

Even so, interns usually spend more time with students than do residents. They can be a great and sympathetic resource, but you should try to understand the pressures they face. Interns will teach you practical aspects of medical care, but when fatigued they often lose interest in disease pathophysiology. Sometimes your intern may be impatient or short-tempered. Don't take it personally.

Residents

Ward teams are usually headed by second-year (or higher) residents who are responsible for supervising interns. Ward residents usually independently interview and examine all patients admitted to their service. They conduct ward rounds and oversee all daily ward activities, but they generally avoid the "scut" work of interns. As team "leaders," residents need to know everything that happens to all team patients. In general, students and interns should clear all management decisions with their residents.

Residents have more time to oversee students, review student notes, and lead didactic sessions. Even so, you may learn information that is more practical from your hands-on interactions with interns.

It is instructive to compare interns and residents in the way they approach patient evaluation and management. Interns generally follow a "shotgun" approach, asking a wide range of routine screening questions, compulsively performing complete physical examinations, collecting a wide battery of routine test results. Interns don't have much experience to draw upon, so they rely on thoroughness. It works quite well. Residents, on the other hand, are considerably more experienced and rely more on acquired instincts than on the brute-force approach of interns. Residents ask focused questions and perform limited physical examinations, yet often manage to unearth more information than do interns, and in less time. Ward residents usually have excellent clinical judgment, even if they are not as knowledgeable as attendings. As a student, your judgment will not be as refined as that of the residents. However, you can be effective on the wards by relying on thoroughness just as interns do.

> Interns rely on thoroughness; Residents rely on judgment.

Specialty Consultants
Sometimes house staff and attendings need additional expertise in the evaluation or management of their patients. In this case, they may ask subspecialty consultants for help.

Teaching hospitals usually have teams available for consultation in subspecialties like infectious diseases, cardiology, and plastic surgery. Just as ward services are led by residents under the supervision of attendings, consult services are usually led by subspecialty **fellows** under the supervision of attendings. Fellows are MD's obtaining subspecialty training after completing residency.

When called for a consult, subspecialty services usually send a student, resident, or fellow to evaluate the patient and present their findings to the consult team. Then the team rounds on the patients with the attending and makes recommendations. Often consult services will continue to follow the patient until the subspecialty problem resolves. Consult services do not usually become primary caretakers. They only make recommendations; it is up to the ward team to decide whether to accept and implement them.

> Have a specific question in mind when you call for consultations.

Have a clear question in mind when you call a subspecialty service for a consult. Otherwise the consultants may not know which problem to address, and their advice may be irrelevant. Never ask the consultant "please evaluate." Ask instead something like, "What is the likelihood this patient has *mesenteric ischemia*?"

Medical Students
The role of medical students on a ward team usually is ill defined. This historically has been a source of great discomfort. Since a MD is ultimately responsible for each patient and often repeats much of the medical student history-taking and examination, the Junior Medical Student may feel superfluous. As a Junior Medical Student, you will find that the more you assume responsibility, lighten the team workload, and become a patient advocate, the less you will feel and seem superfluous. Never feel like an intruder with the team

or with the patient. You have an important mission and a valuable role.

In my opinion, the best way to learn to care for patients is to attempt to function as an intern for a small number of patients: writing all orders and notes, participating in all decisions, performing all procedures. The more you work reliably and thoughtfully, the more you will earn respect and additional attention from the house staff.

> A truly excellent Junior Medical Student aspires to function at the level of an intern.

At the same time, you should study exhaustively every element of the patients' care as issues arise. Reading a textbook is easiest when it is immediately relevant to your patients.

In addition, as a Junior Medical Student, you have more time than anyone else on the team to evaluate and monitor your patients, and to spot important trends everyone else may miss. You also have more time to educate patients about their disease process, compliance, and health maintenance. Patients who have medical students following them in this way are quite lucky.

As a Junior Medical Student, you may not always understand the subtleties of therapeutics, but you certainly are in a position to show compassion and consideration for patients. Be the team member who remembers to draw the curtain around patients being examined during rounds. Be the one who fetches tissues for crying patients and basins for vomiting patients. Be the one who sits down late at night to comfort the frightened.

Though inexperienced at first, you can be your patients' advocate; later, you can become your patients' doctor.

Getting Admitted to the Hospital

Hospital admission is an arduous process for patients.

Many patients are admitted from the emergency department. Small proportions of these patients were in contact (directly or over the telephone) with personal physicians who advised them to go to the ED. The rest have no personal physicians or sensed an emergency, and were taken by ambulance or "walked in" unannounced. Patients register at a desk where they tell a clerk their problem. Their family member, who left to park the car, is lost and has all the important paperwork. A triage nurse measures vital signs and decides how urgently they must be seen by a physician and what initial tests should be done beforehand (*e.g.*, blood tests, ECG, and radiographs). Very ill patients are brought immediately into the patient care area. The remainder wait, often for hours, until staff are available to see them.

At teaching hospitals house officers briefly see the patients and perhaps order additional tests (which require waiting). They discuss their assessment and plan with an attending physician. At this point, a decision is made whether to send the patient home from the ED immediately, whether to treat and observe the patient in the ED, or whether to admit the patient to the hospital. Patients are often surprised and unprepared when advised to stay overnight.

Ideally, patients are sent to the specialty service (*e.g.*, medicine or surgery) that is best equipped to address their main problem. Many have problems overlapping several domains, so it is not always clear where they should be sent. For example, a patient with chronic renal failure and an infected dialysis fistula may be treated by either a medical or a surgical service. Be aware that the decision on which specialty service to send such a patient can be politically charged.

Some patients are admitted directly to the hospital without first visiting the emergency department. Usually these patients already saw their physician and are being admitted "electively" for non-urgent treatment. These may include a brief admission for one of many cycles of immunotherapy, or admission for elective cholecystectomy. Instead of coming to the ED, these patients may go to a separate "admissions" facility, where staff obtain routine blood tests, chest radiographs, and electrocardiograms before sending patients to predetermined specialty services.

Once patients are assigned to a particular location, the medical and nursing staff are notified either by the admissions office or by the emergency department, while they wait to be taken to the appropriate nursing unit by a hospital transporter.

Ideally, the outside physician or ED physician will telephone the admitting house officer and give a brief summary of the patient's problems, extent of diagnostic evaluation completed so far, and relevant past history.

The patient arrives on the floor either with a list of admission tests performed or the ED "sheet," the summary of care received in the ED. Occasionally old medical records are available. The nurse tries to get the patient settled, obtains admission vital signs, tends to IV's, and does an abbreviated H&P.

Eventually the house officer and student get to see the patient. Consecutively or together they perform a detailed history and physical examination as well as procedures like lumbar puncture or blood cultures. Then they write admission orders. More often, the house officer "eyeballs" incoming patients and decides how urgently they need attention. Based on the patient's description by the ED physicians, house officers may write admitting orders after only a cursory evaluation, returning for more careful evaluation after tending to more pressing problems. The JMS evaluation typically will be the most thorough and complete.

Night Call

Somebody needs to be nearby to take care of patient emergencies during the night. At teaching hospitals, interns take turns on **night call**, when they stay overnight at the hospital, take care of new admissions, and take care of current patients with acute problems. Students may take night call as well. Residents on call supervise a number of interns and students. Institutions vary in the frequency of call, the responsibilities of different house officers on call, and the amount of work they need to do on the following day ("post-call").

Spend more time with your patients than you do with your notes.

Students' chief responsibilities during night call are usually to "work-up" (complete a thorough diagnostic evaluation on) a new patient, and write an admission note before going home the next day. Unfortunately, that can distract the JMS from a very exciting time in the hospital — and in my opinion—the best time to learn clinical medicine. The hospital has a skeleton crew at night, yet serious patient management problems keep popping up. Watch your patients and your house officers carefully at night. Nighttime clinical medicine only remotely resembles the material you read in books or discuss with your attendings during daylight hours. In a later section I make personal recommendations about how to get the most out of your night call experiences (See page 134).

Ward Routines from a Patient's Perspective

Hospitals are not restful places. Patients' days are hectic and exhausting. A day may begin at 5:00 a.m. when a respiratory therapist wakes the patient for postural drainage and clapping. A janitor may re-wake the patient at 6:15 while emptying the garbage or mopping the floor. Vital signs may be measured at 7:00. A private attending may visit and examine the patient at 7:20. At 7:45 the intern may come for a visit and examination. The phlebotomist draws morning bloods. Morning medications are given. The nursing staff will help bathe the patient, care for wounds, daily weight, *etc*. Breakfast will arrive. The house staff and medical students will quickly say hello during "work rounds." At 9:00 the patient may be transported to a lab for a special procedure (upper endoscopy or chest radiograph). After lunch, the team resident, the primary intern, and the medical student may make separate lengthy visits. Consulting specialists (*e.g.*, infectious disease, cardiology) may also meet and examine the patient, individually and in subspecialty rounds. Before the afternoon is over, the patient may receive care and replacement of the IV, another phlebotomy, additional medications, another respiratory therapy visit, a trip to occupational therapy, and more laboratory studies. Not only that — the patient is sick!

Try to be sympathetic when your patient tells you he or she is exhausted.

Ward routines from a JMS perspective
Medical students learn by carefully following a small number of patients. A typical day for a Junior Medical Student on an internal medicine or pediatrics service may look like this:

7:20 "Prerounds"

Just like interns, you should review overnight developments on all of your patients each morning. This way you gather up-to-date information for "work rounds" with the rest of your house staff team. It is always embarrassing to learn about an overnight fever *during,* rather than *before,* work rounds. Briefly visit and examine all your patients, record their vital signs, fluid balance, weight, and note overnight fevers. Read the nursing notes about the past shift. Ask the "on call" house officer if there were any problems overnight. Check for results of pending laboratory tests. Finally, check the charts to see if any new orders were written by the "on call" house officer. By the end of prerounds, you should have a list of tasks and plans for the day (See "Master sheets" page 127). You can add to your list during work rounds.

During Prerounds:

Check vital signs.

Record new medications.

Check new developments.

Document latest lab results.

Examine patients.

Prepare a plan for each patient.

8:00 "Work rounds"

In the space of about an hour, the team of residents, interns, and medical students needs to visit every patient on the service, decide how they will be managed that day, and hear formal presentations about new patients who were admitted since the last working rounds. For a two-intern team, this may mean ten new admissions and twenty "old" patients. This amounts to ninety-seconds to see and discuss each old patient and six minutes to see and discuss each new one. Obviously, there is a lot of time-pressure during work rounds.

A common JMS pitfall is to expect too much attention and didactic training during this time. Work rounds can teach you much, but they are designed for patient care more than for JMS training. You will learn that participating in morning management decisions is one of the best ways a house officer or Junior Medical Student can learn. In the meantime, just **listen**.

Work rounds are led by the ward resident. Typically, a team will arrive outside the patient's room. The Junior Medical Student following the patient is expected to make a brief presentation covering any new developments with the patient, vital signs, new physical findings, scheduled diagnostic and therapeutic interventions, and ongoing plans for addressing every problem. (See "Presentations" on page 130). The team will then go to the bedside, the resident will briefly interview and possibly examine the patient, and form a daily plan. Often house officers bring along charts, so they can write new orders as they round.

Plan your day carefully. Use "dead time" to speed patient care.

9:00 Patient care & notes

You may have a short period to see some of your patients before the rest of scheduled morning activities. If you planned your day well during prerounds and work rounds, you can use this short period effectively. It is a good time to draw last-minute bloods, arrange for radiology tests, ask subspecialty consultants to see your patients, *etc*. With your patients "plugged in" for the rest of the morning, more data will be available by the time you are finished with your conferences.

9:30 Attending rounds with students

Attendings will round exclusively with the medical students on the team several times a week. This is a prime learning opportunity. Students generally make formal presentations about the patients they have admitted and are following. Attendings usually take students to the bedside and conduct an interview and physical examination.

10:30 Attending rounds with teams

The rest of the house staff join students at attending rounds. Additional patients are visited and discussed. Usually there are brief lectures.

12:00 Noon conference

On most days there are large didactic sessions for all students and house staff, often with food.

13:00 Student conference

Several times a week larger lectures or seminars are held solely for students. Department heads and chief residents like to hold weekly case discussions.

14:00 Patient care

As you can see, you may not have time actually to take care of your patients until late in the day. This is not a good time to start ordering/collecting routine blood tests, since the results may not be available until evening.

15:00 Radiology and Pathology rounds

Sometime during the afternoon, house staff teams march down to the radiology department and review all new radiographs on their patients. On many teams, it is considered the JMS' responsibility to collect a list of studies to be reviewed from each intern. Interesting pathology specimens may also be reviewed at this time.

15:30 Patient Care

After radiology rounds, the rest of the afternoon is usually left open for the care of patients. Sometimes residents will meet with students for short didactic sessions. They are busy and may forget, so now is a good time to ask for attention.

18:00 Sign-Out

Before going home, every member of the team must do two things: report all new patient developments to the ward resident, and inform the intern "on call" which patients they are responsible for and what problems they can expect overnight. Watch how interns give sign-out to each other; they key-in each other to their patients' most critical problems and contingencies.

How to DO stuff

The Chart Review

While you should try to obtain a complete medical history directly from the patient and family, most patients provide little technical detail. Thoughtful and systematic review of old medical records is an unexpectedly challenging task, but may provide essential information. It should provide detail about ongoing problems, natural history, and past therapy and response. Good chart review also avoids redundant diagnostic tests, particularly dangerous or expensive ones (like cardiac evaluations, magnetic resonance imaging, and biopsy).

Furthermore, your oral presentations frequently fumble unless you have reviewed old records carefully.

> You are "vulnerable" during oral presentations unless you review old charts systematically.

Emergency departments and admissions departments prioritize patient "flow" over medical records. But it is essential to assemble current and past medical records when patients arrive on the floor. Do not delay contacting outside institutions and physicians to obtain relevant outpatient notes, admission notes, discharge summaries, and test results read over the phone, faxed, or emailed to you.

Here are some important parts of the chart you should check:

- **Discharge summary**

  This is usually a typed narrative of the patient's problems and hospital course. Regard discharge summaries with skepticism, since important details are often omitted or glossed over.

- **Admission note**

  This contains details about the patient's presentation and complete physical examination. Beware of the assessments, which may change during the hospital course.

- **Consult sheets**

  These reflect "expert opinions" on specific problems. You need to hunt them out specifically, since they are usually buried in the chart. Know that consultants' opinions also change over time, so you should check their ongoing comments in the progress notes.

- **Operative notes**

  These describe indications, procedures, and findings.

- **Pathology reports**

  On surgical specimens, for example, report what histopathology revealed or, for example, whether surgical margins were free of tumor.

- **Laboratory tests**

  Tests from the past are often relevant to the patient's current problems, including blood tests, electrocardiograms, radiology reports. These help you identify interval changes.

- **Discharge medications and follow-up plans**

  Make sure to find out if there have been changes in medications since discharge.

- **Progress notes**

  These usually have important details omitted from discharge summaries. Skim these sections, at least. If you have time or unanswered questions, skim through the orders and vital sign sheets as well.

- **The patient**

  Don't forget that the **patient** or family can clarify questions raised by the chart.

Ask the patient for help when you are confused!

Your chart review should be specifically tailored to the problem list. A few examples follow:

- **Ischemic heart disease**

    Identify cardiac risk factors, previous infarctions or vascular disease, tests of cardiac function, anatomy, and therapy. Include past level of function (*e.g.*, angina after walking 200 feet), results of electrocardiograms, exercise tests, nuclear medicine studies, echocardiograms, cardiac catheterization, details of prior cardiac interventions or surgery, and medications.

- **Diabetes mellitus**

    Identify progression of end-organ disease and "tightness" of glucose control. For example, find funduscopic exams, renal function, blood sugars, glycohemoglobin, insulin requirements, evidence of neuropathy or vasculopathy.

- **Colonic neoplasm**

    Describe any surgery, pathology reports, evidence of metastases and surgical stage, tumor markers, weight loss, *etc.*

- **Chronic obstructive lung disease**

    Past serial pulmonary function tests, arterial blood gases, chest radiographs, infections, evidence of right-sided heart disease, past medications.

- **Chronic renal insufficiency**

    Include serial BUN, creatinine, and creatinine clearance results, blood pressure control, and etiology of renal impairment, if known.

- **Infections**

    Note the source of infection, the specimens obtained, the organisms isolated and their antibiotic sensitivities, the antibiotics used and the duration of treatment, the clinical response and time to defervesce.

- **Obstetrics patients**

Identify past OB risks like pregnancy-induced hypertension or pregnancy-induced diabetes, sexually-transmitted disease, immunizations, Rh, *etc.*

- **Psychiatric patients**

    Past medications, response, side-effects. Make sure past diagnoses (especially schizophrenia and borderline personality) are substantiated.

Chart Lore

> Avoid "chart lore:" Substantiate past diagnoses.

Spurious information sometimes enters patients' medical records and never leaves. For example, does the patient really have asthma or chronic obstructive pulmonary disease? Did the patient really have a "heart attack?"

Orders

Purpose of orders

Since physicians order, but don't actually deliver most hospital care, parameters of patient care must be carefully described in orders for the rest of the health care team. Physician orders convey a lot of information:

- Why the patient was admitted.

- Who are the responsible physicians.

- What is the patient's condition and what is the likelihood of sudden deterioration.

- What should nurses monitor and reasons they should immediately contact house officers.

- Routine contingency plans for which house officers need not be contacted ("PRN" orders).

- Limitations on a patient's daily life (*e.g.* activity, diet, visitors, *etc.*).

- Hazards of care, both to staff and to patient (*e.g.*, allergy, infection risk, immunocompromise).

- Circumstances when emergency care should not be offered (*e.g.*, Do not resuscitate orders).

> Truly excellent Junior Medical Students write all of the orders on their patients.

Several kinds of orders will be described below. Admission orders, which usually are the most extensive, will be covered in most detail. Similar orders are written postoperatively and when patients are transferred between nursing units or medical services. Special orders are also written when patients are discharged from the hospital.

How orders are written & processed

Electronic order entry has been adopted worldwide. Take the time to learn old-fashioned manual order entry, so that you are ready for computer "downtimes" and so that you understand all that is necessary for basic inpatient care.

> Illegible handwriting is more dangerous than you think. Secretaries who have limited medical training transcribe your orders.

Medication Summaries (aka Medical Treatment Records, MTRs) are guidebooks for each patient which list all medication and nursing orders. Whenever a drug is administered, a notation is left in the MTR for confirmation. At the beginning of each nursing shift, nurses review the MTRs on their patients and schedule the tasks they must perform (including drug administrations) for that shift. MTRs are also a good place to look when you are reviewing an old chart for medications actually given to a patient.

Writing Admission orders

Contemporary order-entry systems are algorithm-driven. Learn the internal logic of these pre-planned orders, but do not become dependent on them. Otherwise you may not be able to function during electronic "downtimes."

Admission orders to a nonsurgical service are the most extensive. The most popular format follows the acronym "ADCA VAN DIMLS," for Admit, Diagnosis, Condition, Allergy, Vital signs, Activity, Nursing, Diet, IV fluids, Medications, Labs, and Special.

> Remember:
> ADCA VAN DIMLS
> - or -
> ADC VANDALISM

Admit
This is the formal authorization to admit a patient to a specific medical service or nursing unit. Usually this order includes the contact info of the intern and/or attending.

> Example:
> *Admit to Oncology Unit Tower 6 / Dr. Armitage #216-999-9999.*

Diagnosis
Although the patient has not yet been evaluated thoroughly, you must list the reason for admission or the working diagnosis. Include important secondary diagnoses. Do not abbreviate, since you are also writing for non-medical personnel.

> Example:
> *Diagnosis: Pneumonia (possibly tuberculosis), congestive heart failure, diabetes mellitus.*

Condition
Sometimes a patient looks pretty good but is in fact very sick. Here you can convey that to the staff. In describing the seriousness of

illness, this line helps the nurses tune in to the psychosocial needs of the patient and family. Typically, hospital staff may release patients' condition when callers inquire by name.

Possibilities include critical (in which case they usually belong in an intensive care unit), serious (which includes hemodynamic instability), stable or fair, good, and undetermined.

> Example:
> Condition: serious.

Allergy

> A truly excellent Junior Medical Student carefully documents (in notes) the specific medication, condition, timing, clinical response, and treatment of all hypersensitivity reactions.

Include allergies (hypersensitivity reactions) and other adverse reactions to medications, food, bandage tape, etc. This information usually gets plastered all over the patient, the chart, and the MTR in an attempt to avoid administration, usually by an unfamiliar physician. "NKDA" means "no known drug allergy."

> Examples:
> Allergy: NKDA.
>
> -or-
>
> Allergy: penicillin (anaphylaxis), povidone-iodine (eczema).

Declaring an allergy can mean forever condemning a patient to suboptimal therapy, for example, avoidance of beta-lactam antimicrobials in life-threatening infections. Make sure you carefully describe in your notes the allergic response, and make sure you are right! Distinguish allergic reactions, which may be life threatening, from benign "drug intolerance" or side effects, like constipation or rash, or from coincidence. Note that "allergy" to specific narcotics raises concerns over narcotic-seeking behavior.

Vital signs

Here is where you specify how often and how carefully a patient should be monitored. Vital signs are among the most valuable components of physical exams, and are easy to obtain. Obviously, patients need careful and frequent monitoring when they are most unstable, for example, after surgery and invasive procedures, during medical emergencies like diabetic ketoacidosis, severe pneumonia, etc.

> *Examples:*
> *Vital signs every 8 hours.*
> *Vital signs hourly x 4 then every two hours x 4 then q shift.*
> *Neuro checks every two hours x 8h then every four hours x 8h then discontinue.*
> *Postural VS each morning.*
> *Weight daily x 4d then every other day*
> *Record inputs and outputs.*
> *Call house officer for T > 38.5°C.*

Know that monitoring beyond the nursing routine (which consists ordinarily of temperature, pulse, blood pressure, and respiratory rate measured once per shift) can be difficult for short-staffed nursing teams. When patients need nursing care beyond what can reasonably be provided by a floor team, the patient belongs in an intensive-care setting. Out of courtesy to the nurses, if you are ordering intensive monitoring, try to specify endpoints and discontinue the monitoring as soon as possible.

Weighing patients can be very difficult for nursing staff, but weight trends are so valuable for assessing volume status that it is worth your insistence. A record of fluid balance (enteral and parenteral inputs, urine, stool, and drainage outputs) can guide therapy, but is often inaccurate. Postural (orthostatic) vital sign determinations are often helpful as well.

You can specify that nurses should contact you for certain vital signs (many people write this under the "Specials" section below). Nurses may be insulted if you ask them to notify you for SBP < 80, but sometimes the info is collected by nursing aides who may not recognize the urgency. Check this out in advance.

26...How to DO stuff   Truly Excellent Junior Medical Student

> **A respiratory rate of 20 is abnormal.**

The myth that a normal respiratory rate is 20 per minute provides an easy way to know whether your patients' respiratory rates are truly measured. If your patient consistently has a RR of 20, you can be fairly sure the values are fudged.

Activity

Here you specify what the patient is permitted to do. For example, patients with balance or gait disorders should walk only with assistance, especially if they are at risk for fracture. Patients with wounds that may dehisce should not be permitted to leave their beds. Patients with peripheral cellulitis or edema should have the affected extremity elevated. Patients with reflux esophagitis or CHF should have the head of bed elevated. Patients who endanger their wounds or vital catheters may need to be restrained under appropriate conditions. Recovering patients should be forced out of bed and encouraged to walk. The superior JMS will be on hand to witness and assist reluctant walkers. The obvious first destination for walking patients is the bathroom, and if that is too far, the patient should have a bedside commode.

> *Examples:*
> *Activity: ad libitum (or just "ad lib").*
> *- or -*
> *Bed rest (specify strict / bathroom privileges).*
> *- or -*
> *Dangle legs over side of bed in AM, up in chair in PM and three times daily thereafter.*
> *Walk with assistance four times daily.*
> *Elevate head of bed 30°.*
> *Seizure precautions.*
> *Overhead trapeze.*

Nursing

Here you order additional monitoring parameters and specific nursing interventions not already mentioned. Possible measurements include: calorie counts; fingerstick glucose determination; urine dipstick for glucose, ketones, protein, and specific gravity; stool guaiac testing; nasogastric suction output for guaiac and pH; postural vital signs; or abdominal girth.

Some interventions include postural drainage and clapping for patients who have impaired clearance of respiratory secretions or atelectasis; wound and dressing care orders; decubitus care; special beds; incentive spirometry; enemas; antigravity stockings; nasogastric tube for intermittent suction; Foley catheter to be placed and left to continuous drainage; bladder irrigation and post-void residual bladder volume; bedside commode; cooling blanket; patient hygiene; isolation or protection for infection or immunocompromise.

> Examples:
> Glucometer before each meal and at bedtime.
> Guaiac all stools.
> Urine ketones each shift x 24h.
> Respiratory therapist for PD&C four times daily.
> Thigh-high Thrombo-Embolic Deterrent (TED) Hose
> Respiratory isolation for possible tuberculosis.
> Air-mattress bed.
> Elevate right foot 20°.
> Sacral decubitus care, including saline wet to dry dressing three times daily.

Diet

A patient's gotta eat. Here you specify the consistency, content, quantity, and means of delivery. In healthy people, just order the greasy "house diet."

> Example:
> Diet: 1500 kCal, soft mechanical, renal, ADA.
> NPO after midnight.
> Hold breakfast tray and restore diet on return from upper endoscopy.

Adults who face possible general or moderate anesthesia are kept NPO (no oral intake) approximately four-eight hours before the procedure to reduce the risk of aspiration from respiratory failure or endotracheal intubation. Know that patients who have undergone surgical procedures often have a transient paresis of the GI tract after surgery ("postop ileus") and are at risk for intestinal obstruction if you feed them solid food too early. After evidence that bowel motility has returned (*e.g.*, flatus and bowel sounds), postoperative patients are offered low-bulk food and their diet is advanced as tolerated.

Have mercy on hungry patients. If a patient will undergo a simple procedure in the morning for which they have been kept NPO, ask that the breakfast tray be held until their return. If a surgical procedure is canceled or postponed, renew a patient's dietary orders promptly.

Consistency
Clear-liquids. Refers to residue-free liquids like broth, tea, jello, strained juice. These are nutritionally inadequate but better than nothing.

Full-liquids. Refers to easily-digestible food that is liquid at room temperature, including ice cream, cream soups, strained meats. This diet can be used for a long time.

Soft diet. Food that is easily chewed and digested but with no seasonings and minimal bulk.

Soft mechanical. A normal diet for edentulous patients.

Content
ADA (American Dietetic Association) diet of polyunsaturated fats and complex carbohydrates for patients with diabetes mellitus.

Renal diet (low-protein, low potassium & other electrolytes) for patients with renal insufficiency.

Low-sodium, for patients with CHF, ascites, cirrhosis, *etc.* Note that a **"No added salt"** diet is equivalent to a **"2 gram sodium"** diet or about 4g salt; it generally means no salt is added during food preparation. More intensive salt restriction makes food especially unpalatable and expensive to prepare.

Low-protein (for hepatic failure, renal insufficiency).

Lactose-restricted (for lactase-deficient patients).

Gluten-free (for suspected gluten-sensitive enteropathy).

Low-tyramine (for patients on MAO inhibitors).

Kosher or **vegetarian** when appropriate.

Quantity
Specify caloric restriction or "liberal" for all-you-can-eat type behavior. Ask the dietitian for help in determining the degree of caloric restriction or supplement.

Delivery
Via Dobhoff-type feeding tube, when necessary. A discussion of forced enteral feeding and of parenteral nutrition is beyond the scope of this guide.

Pre-Procedure feeding
One of the great ways for a medical student to interfere with medical care is to neglect to plan for surgical or invasive procedures. Don't forget to keep patients *NPO* before procedures that might risk aspiration of gastric contents. The procedure schedules may be full, so inadvertently feeding patients can dramatically prolong their hospital stay or harm their care.

Intravenous Fluids
Here you specify the type and volume of IV fluids you want administered, as well as care of the IV catheter. A good discussion of fluid and electrolyte management is beyond the scope of this guide, but here are some pointers.

> Avoid continuous IV fluid orders; instead specify endpoints and reevaluate.

IV fluids are as dangerous as any other medication; fluid overload is one of the most common iatrogenic diseases. Make sure that there are clear indications for fluid infusion. Be especially careful with debilitated, elderly, or very young patients. One way to avoid inadvertent fluid overload is to avoid the common practice of writing continuous orders for IV fluids. Always specify endpoints (time or volume) after which you should re-evaluate and re-order fluids if necessary.

IV cannulas clot quickly if fluid is not flowing through them constantly or if they are not flushed periodically. Make sure that your IV orders do not expire before the last bag runs out; otherwise, the IV may clot and you may need to start a new one. You can order IV fluid at a low rate (KVO or "keep vein open"), but beware that this amounts to 200-500mL/day of fluid, which may be too much in a volume-sensitive patient. When IV fluids are not running, you should order routine saline lock (aka *HepLock*) flushes, meaning that every few hours the IV catheter will be flushed with saline or with dilute heparin solution.

On medical services, intravenous fluids given to compensate for inadequate oral intake usually consist of three components:

Dextrose

Since plain water will destroy veins by virtue of being hypotonic, a modest amount of sugar is added when you want to instill free water into patients. When saline solution is infused, dextrose is not needed to protect veins; however since patients requiring IV fluids usually have inadequate oral intake, a small amount of dextrose (almost) never hurts. 5% dextrose (abbreviated D5) is nearly isotonic, approximately 300 mM. Junior nurses are sometimes concerned about infusing dextrose into patients with diabetes mellitus; you can reassure them that the relatively small amount of dextrose is usually inconsequential, even in patients with diabetes.

Saline

> Use modest volumes of saline in patients with congestive heart failure.

Isotonic (or "normal" or 0.9%) saline is infused in patients who are intravascularly volume depleted and cannot immediately make up these needs by drinking. If they are not volume depleted and need free water more than they need salt, lower concentrations of saline are infused (e.g., normal saline half-diluted in water). Isotonic saline is 0.9% sodium chloride in water, 154 mM. ½ NS is 0.45% sodium chloride in water. Patients with congestive heart failure quickly become volume-overloaded when given saline infusions.

Potassium

> Don't add K^+ to IV fluids until you know the patient's kidney function.

Patients receiving IV fluids often become hypokalemic if they don't receive supplemental potassium. Both hypo- and hyper-kalemia are extremely dangerous yet common iatrogenic conditions. A small amount of potassium (e.g., 10-20 mEq/liter) is usually added to maintenance IV fluids, but not unless their renal function is known to be intact. Patients with renal insufficiency may quickly become hyperkalemic if they are given IV potassium. Drugs such as spironolactone and ACE inhibitors also will cause hyperkalemia with injudicious supplements.

Hospitals have begun requiring automated intravenous pump control, and restricted amounts and rates for parenteral potassium administrations. Oral or enteral routes are preferred.

Intravenous fluids are usually given for one of two indications:

Volume resuscitation

When patients are intravascularly volume-depleted, as during severe dehydration or hemorrhage, IV fluids are given to fill their blood vessels. Since free-water has a larger volume of distribution than do salt or colloid solutions, only the latter are used for resuscitation of volume-depleted patients. Typically, isotonic salt solutions are used. "Normal" or isotonic saline or the surgical cocktail "lactated Ringers" are examples.

Dextrose solutions are not very helpful in volume resuscitation. As soon as dextrose is infused, it is rapidly metabolized leaving only free water in the intravascular space. The free water quickly moves out of blood vessels into tissue; yet only intravascular volume, not tissue water, is hemodynamically important.

Maintenance Fluids

> Maintenance fluids:
> - 100mL/kg/day for the first 10 kg.
> - 50mL/kg/day for the second 10 kg.
> - 20mL/kg/day for the remainder.
> - Subtract oral intake from total.
> - Increase for fever or surgery.
> - Reduce for CHF.

Patients who have inadequate oral intake (e.g., due to surgery or nausea) may become dehydrated from urination and perspiration unless they receive maintenance IV fluids. Since these patients are not (yet) intravascularly volume-depleted, they usually do not need as much salt as do patients being volume-resuscitated. Typically, they are given a mixture of dextrose, salt in hypotonic concentrations, and potassium to make up for their reduced eating and their continued urination.

Medications

A discussion of how to order and prescribe medications is provided in detail later in this book. (See section on medications, page 37)

Briefly, you should specify the drug, the dose, the frequency, the mode of delivery, and any special instructions. Note any medications the patient ingested prior to admission.

Labs

Here you order laboratory tests. Again, note any lab tests which may have been taken upon hospital admission. Body fluid specimens are collected and submitted by the nursing staff. You should ask that additional specimens be held for your own laboratory fun: Gram stain, culture plating, urinalysis, fecal leukocytes, *etc*. Routine phlebotomy is available at most hospitals, and ward secretaries usually fill out the necessary requisitions.

For other studies you may have to fill out the requisition or call and schedule the procedure yourself. Notify the ward secretary of scheduled procedures so that the patient won't be allowed off the floor at that time.

Special

This section is for everything you haven't written so far. Requests for special technician intervention or for special therapy can be included here. Parameters for nurses to call you can also be put here (See Vital Signs above). Unlike nurses on surgical services, nurses on medical services may resent being told to call for abnormal vital signs.

> *Examples:*
>
> *Respiratory therapist to induce sputum for bacterial culture.*
> *Call HO for DBP < 50 or SBP < 90 or SBP > 180 or HR > 130 or RR < 8 or T > 38.5.*
> *Physical therapy (req in front).*

Routine patient orders

You will probably have to enter additional orders or discontinue previous ones throughout your patient's hospital stay. It is best to review the medication treatment summary and add routine orders at the same time you write the daily progress note. Keep track of the current medications ordered for your patient.

If you are changing the dose of a medication, be sure to use a word like "change," or else the patient may inadvertently receive additional doses of the same medication. It is important that you include the date and time for every order you write. Other members of the team may need this information to decipher the events of the day.

> *Example:*
> *5/8/2020 14:00*
> *Change gentamicin to 110 mg IV q8°.*
> *Discontinue vancomycin.*

Writing discharge orders

Discharges must be planned in advance, even though most patients want to leave the hospital immediately. Patients need to be instructed on how to care for themselves, how to take their medications, and to watch for specific warning signs. All patients should be scheduled for a follow-up appointment and given a telephone number of a nurse or physician they can call with problems. (Remember that the hospital stay is only one component of their health care.)

Discharge orders have a broad target audience. Nurses, who in general take the most time instructing patients, need to know what the post-discharge care entails. Sometimes patients return to the emergency department soon after discharge with problems related to their hospital stay; discharge orders provide a quick summary of current illness and therapy. Finally, the orders permit the staff and administration to anticipate the availability of an empty bed for new patients. The discharge orders follow a general format:

Discharge
Authorizes the discharge at a certain time. In general, patients are discharged to the care/responsibility of an adult, *e.g.*, "Discharge home with wife."

Diagnosis
The primary reason for hospital stay, which often is different from the admitting diagnosis. Here you are writing for the benefit of the harried emergency department physician.

Medications
Usually you have to write individual prescriptions for discharge medications. This "order" is written to document these medications for the instructing nurse and for the ED physician (should the patient return). List them as you would for regular orders. If the patient will be tapering a medication (*e.g.*, gradually reducing doses of a corticosteroid), record the taper schedule here.

Follow-up
Write whom the patient will see and when, and try to include the telephone number. If necessary, order that an appointment be scheduled.

> Example:
> 3/15/2020 17:30

Discharge patient in AM after she is seen by HO.
Diagnosis: Pneumonia
Medications:
Amoxicillin 500mg po q8h x 7d.
Atenolol 50mg po qd.
Docusate sodium 100mg po bid.
F/U: Dr. Khalaf at general medicine clinic 3/21/2020 at 13:15.

> Make sure your patient has follow-up arrangements before discharge.

Final tips on orders:

Orders written by medical students are not processed until they are countersigned by a physician. This can cause needless delay.

Once you are on good terms with various interns and residents, they may start to countersign your orders without reading them. If they do, they are doing you and your patient a disservice. Even though you should have thought carefully about everything you have written, sometimes there is something wrong or inappropriate in your orders. Discussing your orders is a good learning opportunity as well. Forged countersignatures or password-sharing can lead to hospital disciplinary action. Don't do it.

> Don't let house officers countersign your orders blindly.

Urgent orders

Some interventions are urgent. Orders marked stat or now take priority over all other nursing tasks, and are expected to be implemented immediately.

> Notify nurses personally when you write stat orders.

You must notify nurses that you have written an urgent order, either personally or via the division secretary.

Note that laboratories and the pharmacy have a more liberal interpretation of the word "stat." If you need a lab test performed immediately, you should deliver the specimen to the lab and talk to the technician personally. If you need a drug or blood product immediately and it is not available on the floor, you or a nurse should talk directly to a pharmacist or staff of the blood bank. You may prefer to deliver especially precious specimens personally; would you want a messenger to transport your cerebrospinal fluid?

> A truly excellent Junior Medical Student delivers important specimens and picks up urgent drugs.

Review the Medication Summary

You should frequently review the Medication Summary on your patients. Sometimes an important treatment has been withheld or refused, and the Medication Summary may be the only indication of this fact. The Medication Summary is the only record that PRN medications have been administered. Check the Medication Summary also for accurate transcription of new orders, for duplicate orders, potential adverse drug interactions, and orders that are no longer necessary. Try to discontinue special nursing orders, like frequent weights, vital signs, and chem-stix, which require much nursing effort but no longer are necessary. Sometimes important orders to treat (or not-to-treat) expire and are automatically discontinued without your knowledge. You may find many surprises in the Medication Summary, especially when other house officers are writing orders on your patients in your absence.

Every few days the progress note should include an updated list of drugs from the Medication Summary.

Write unambiguously

Many free-text orders are ambiguous when scrutinized. Sometimes the nurse will try to "read your mind," and carry out the order, though not necessarily as you intended. Otherwise, the nurse or ward secretary may page you for clarification. Even attention-starved Junior Medical Students quickly tire when called frequently to clarify orders. Finally, be sure to specify the time and date whenever you write an order in the chart.

Avoidable disasters
- Writing orders on the wrong patient's chart.
- Ordering drugs at the wrong dosage or frequency. This often happens when you rely on other people's wrong information. Always check drug doses in a reputable source before writing for them (The National Library of Medicine USA *Dailymed* https://dailymed.nlm.nih.gov/ is a good source).
- Failure to notify nurses directly of urgent orders.
- Forgetting to sign/countersign orders.
- Writing ambiguous or illegible orders.

Medications & Prescriptions

Junior Medical Students spend the bulk of their time on medical services learning to perform a thorough diagnostic evaluation. At this stage of training it is easy to lose sight of the fact that patients are evaluated in an attempt to choose proper therapy. In attempting medical therapy, many JMSs forget important principles, which I will mention here only briefly.

All therapeutic maneuvers should have clearly-defined objectives, anticipated measures of response to therapy, ongoing diagnostic alternatives, and attempts to minimize risk of iatrogenic illness. For example, in treating a presumed pneumonia, the objectives are to eradicate the infection and improve the patient's outcome. The specific steps would be:

- Obtain a diagnostic specimen (sputum Gram stain and culture).
- Attempt to eradicate the most likely organisms (with relatively broad-spectrum antibiotics).
- Once a specific pathogen is isolated, consider switching to narrower-spectrum antimicrobials for better efficacy and to reduce selection pressure for resistant organisms.

- Follow the patient's symptoms, vital signs, physical exam, blood counts, and chest radiograph as indices of clinical response.
- Observe the patient carefully for evidence of drug toxicity, and for the possibility that the illness represents not the presumptive diagnosis of pneumonia but instead another process, for example a vasculitis. The latter may appear more likely if the clinical response is poor even though the therapy is judged adequate for the pneumonia.

Medications should be ordered only after clear therapeutic endpoints and clinical indices have been established, with the full knowledge that they are potentially toxic and possibly inappropriate.

Writing medication orders
Medication orders consist of the drug name, the dose, the frequency of administration, the mode of delivery, and any special instructions.

Time and date
Specify these for every order you write. The information is important for staff, for quality control and occasionally for consulting physicians.

Drug name
Write the generic name of the drug, without abbreviations. It is bad form to use brand names, even though it is common practice. It is also very difficult to remember two or more names for each drug. Worse, abbreviations can lead to catastrophic misinterpretations. For example, the common abbreviation MSO4 is sometimes used to mean morphine sulfate, and at other times refers to magnesium sulfate.

Use generic drug names.
Avoid abbreviations.

Drug dose
Specify the dose and units of measurement. Do not rely exclusively on patients or on nursing notes to remember the correct dose of drugs when you are continuing drugs patients were taking outside

the hospital. Check their actual prescription bottles or contact their pharmacist or private physician. Check a reputable guide to make sure the dose is correct. Be aware of special circumstances when you need to alter drug dosages (e.g., renal insufficiency, hepatic disease, or interacting drugs. Be sure to check drug doses in patients with renal or hepatic failure.

> Verify correct doses.
> Adjust dose appropriately for impaired drug clearance or drug interactions.

Frequency of administration

Specify a schedule. Latin abbreviations are common and historically relevant, but nowadays medical centers require you to use whole words.

Latin Prescription Dosing:	Required Non-abbreviated English-language Dosing Schedule:
q.d.	Each day
q.o.d.	Every other day
b.i.d.	Twice daily during waking hours
t.i.d.	Three times daily during waking hours
q.i.d.	Four times daily during waking hours
q.6h	Every six hours
q.H.S.	At bedtime
q.A.C.	Before each meal

Note that the "t.i.d." and "q 8 hours" are not synonymous: the former means three times a day during waking hours (which may amount to every six hours), while the latter means exactly every eight hours. When some variation in blood concentration is acceptable, "t.i.d." is preferable, since patients are then permitted to sleep through the night.

Route of delivery

Specify the route by which the drug should be administered. Common abbreviations are listed in the chart below. Again, write complete English words if there is any possibly confusion.

Latin Common Abbreviation	Required Non-Abbreviated Prescription Routes of Delivery
p.o.	Orally
p.r.	Per rectum
per N.G.	By nasogastric tube
S.L.	Sublingual
I.V.	Intravenous
O.D.	Right eye
O.S.	Left eye
O.U.	Both eyes

Examples:
3/15/2020 09:15
Furosemide 40 mg p.o. daily, first dose in AM.
Beclomethasone inhaler 2 puffs qid via spacer.
Gentamicin 120 mg IV loading dose STAT then 80 mg IV q 8h. Please call HO to draw trough and peak levels around third dose.
Isosorbide dinitrate 20 mg po three times daily given q6h.
Captopril 6.25 mg po three times daily. Measure BP q 30 min x 2 after first dose. Hold subsequent doses if systolic BP < 100mm.

PRN medications

PRN, which means "as needed," provides a contingency plan for medications to be given at patient request and/or nursing discretion. PRN orders are commonly written for analgesics, hypnotics, and laxatives.

"Clever" house officers or JMSs write many PRN orders to minimize "annoying" nursing calls in the middle of the night. Unfortunately, in distancing yourself further from the hour-to-hour management of patients, you may not be aware of important new problems as they arise. For example, analgesic/antipyretics (like acetaminophen) may mask fevers. While it may be good to anticipate minor problems that don't demand your immediate attention, it is not good to put your patients entirely on "auto-pilot."

Make sure you check Medication Summaries regularly when you have written for PRN medications. You may find important trends. For example, the nurses may not tell you that a patient has asked for much more morphine in the past few days.

Pediatric medications

Since children vary in size their drug doses are adjusted for weight or body surface area. Pediatric drug orders usually include the specific dose as well as the dose per kilogram of child. This practice reduces errors.

> Example:
> *Amoxicillin 100 mg (10 mg/kg) po q 8h.*

Writing Prescriptions

Prescriptions are drug orders for outpatient medications, to be filled by an outside pharmacist. They differ from in-house drug orders in an important way: the patient is responsible for obtaining and administering the drug. Since nurses won't be supervising drug administration, you should leave concise patient instructions on the prescription. Prescriptions follow a standard format, including:

- Hospital/physician identification. A pharmacist may need to contact you for clarification.
- Patient identification, including hospital number and date of birth if necessary.
- Date
- Drug name.

- Drug preparation (*e.g.,* tablets & size) and dose. Some pharmacies expect you to specify exactly what size pills you want.
- Frequency of administration.
- Quantity to dispense.
- Instructions to place on label (optional).
- Refills. For some medications, patients can take the same prescription back to the pharmacy for refills without seeing you first.

Example:
March 15, 2020   John Doe   Hosp #123 456
5 Main St, Anytown USA

Rx: Furosemide 40 mg tablets.
Disp: Sixty.
Sig: Take one tablet by mouth each morning. "Water pill."
Refills: None.
 Signed,

Shorthand version:
3/15/2020
Furosemide 40 mg 1 po qAM #60.
No refills.
 Signed,

Bear in mind
- Quantities of pills to dispense and of numbers of refills are best written as words, to prevent alteration.
- The number of tablets taken each dose are usually written as italicized roman numerals.
- Most states and medical centers regulate controlled substances (*e.g.,* narcotics and benzodiazepines) prescriptions and dispensation. Physicians may be required to check statewide Prescription Drug Monitoring Program registries for controlled substances before prescribing opioids

for chronic pain, may be required to use special prescription pads, and may not be permitted to allow refills.

- Try to include the indication for the medication in the signa section (*e.g.,* "for headache"), in terms the patient can understand. This reminds the patient, the family, and the emergency department doctor.

How to Learn about Drugs

For economy, hospitals maintain a limited formulary of drugs routinely available. This also makes pharmacology easier for the clinician, since representatives of each class of drugs are chosen for the formulary rather than a bewildering variety of "me-too" products. For example, a hospital may make available the H2-antagonist ranitidine, but not famotidine, or nizatidine. Similarly, the ureidopenicillin mezlocillin may be on formulary, but not azlocillin or piperacillin.

> Know "everything" about each drug your patients take.

As a JMS you should approach drugs first as broad classes rather than as individual agents. For example, when prescribing an afterload-reducing agent, concentrate on the broad hemodynamic effects of this category before focusing on the particulars of hydralazine, nitroprusside, or ACE inhibitors. Moreover, when learning about ACE inhibitors, don't bother distinguishing between captopril, enalapril, and lisinopril; learn about the one on formulary and consider the others to be similar. Read about the broad classes of drugs in textbooks of pharmacology.

On admission, your patients probably will need to continue a number of medications taken at home. Don't blindly reorder the same list of drugs. Instead, take advantage of this medication reconciliation to review thoroughly the patient's drug therapy and to consider whether they really need each drug. As a JMS you are responsible for knowing "everything" about the drugs you prescribe for your patients, including the mode of action, common side-effects, serious adverse reactions, drug interactions, modes of elimination, and contraindications.

Laxatives for Total Bowel Control

Bowel movements are an important part of the day for most patients. But many common hospital measures make patients constipated, including bedrest, analgesics, psychiatric drugs, certain antacids, and verapamil. Total bowel control should be one of your goals on the wards. Here a stepwise approach:

- Prophylaxis with bulk-forming agents. Except for those at risk for intestinal obstruction, I put all of my patients on prophylactic psyllium preparations (*e.g.*, Metamucil brand) to increase fecal mass and soften stools. Bulk forming agents don't take effect for one or more days.

> "Metamucil" one or two tablespoons in 250mL fluid twice a day prevents constipation in most patients.

- Prophylactic or PRN stool softening surfactants also are very benign. They usually take effect in a day or two. Docusate sodium (Colace or Surfak brands) is a common preparation.

> Docusate sodium 100mg po bid can be used concurrently with psyllium as prophylaxis.

- Irritant suppositories can be used sparingly if you need immediate action. Bisacodyl 10mg suppositories (*Dulcolax* brand), causes stooling in 15 to 60 minutes. Prolonged use of irritant suppositories is not recommended, so you should only order single doses.

> Bisacodyl suppository 1 per rectum, used sparingly, can succeed when a trial of docusate sodium fails.

- Osmotic agents are alternatives to irritants and can be used in otherwise healthy patients who can take drugs orally. Magnesium hydroxide suspension (Milk of Magnesia) 30mL is well tolerated and used very commonly. Magnesium citrate, 1 bottle po, will cause an even brisker catharsis. Note that osmotic agents can be absorbed (and are therefore contraindicated in patients with renal insufficiency or CHF) or can cause dehydration. Magnesium citrate should be given to patients just after undergoing barium enema, since the barium may cause fecal impaction if not immediately expelled from the bowel.

> Milk of magnesia is contraindicated in patients with renal insufficiency.

- Enemas sometimes help where other agents fail. Fleets is a popular brand of buffered saline and phosphate. Tap water and mineral oil enemas are less gentle alternatives.

All laxatives are relatively contraindicated in patients with cramps, nausea, or vomiting which may reflect undiagnosed surgical disease.

Wash your hands and instruments

All surfaces at medical centers are likely contaminated with pathogens, some of them quite dangerous to your patients. This includes your hands, your stethoscope, your mobile phone or notepad, your clothing, and your shoes.

Imagine everything and everyone coated with permanent ink.

Please be sure to wash your hands before and after every medical encounter. Show your patients that you are doing so.

Writing Notes

Admission Notes

Every newly-admitted patient undergoes a painstaking diagnostic evaluation, including some routine and some special tests. By following standard protocols, even the most inexperienced JMS can perform a thorough initial diagnostic evaluation. The fruit of your evaluation is an admission note.

The admission note should not be a tedious record of the serial progression of your thoughts. Instead it should be planned carefully, leading the reader to the results of the evaluation as outlined at the end in the problem list, differential diagnosis, and plan.

Each sentence should address the questions raised in the end by your problem list. If for example you list dyspnea, fever, and productive cough as problems, then the "history of present illness" section of your admission note should include the answer to every question you would ask to distinguish pneumonia from other processes like congestive heart failure or obstructive pulmonary disease.

When you get more daring, you can include "red-herrings" in your admission note to try to lead your supervisors away from a less obvious diagnosis.

Writing the admission note
Here I review only the skeleton, with some comments.

Title, Date, Time, Patient Name & Hospital Number

Informants
Indicate how you got your information: from the patient, nursing home attendants, old hospital records, parents, children, the private physician, *etc*. If they seem unreliable, say so.

Reason for admission
This may be more informative than a chief complaint. A patient may complain of nausea but may be admitted because of diabetic ketoacidosis. In as few words as possible, mention both in this

section. Be sure to include duration of complaint. Detail the complaints in the next section.

History of the present illness (HPI)

Identify the patient, age, sex, and ethnic background, if relevant. In a short sentence, mention relevant underlying conditions. Describe the symptoms and progression as you were taught in physical diagnosis.

Most HPI's are best structured in chronological order, from the time of onset of the problem requiring admission. Either record time relative to the time of admission (*e.g.*, hours, days, or months prior to admission) or using calendar dates. Do not mix both. Do not use relative dates (*e.g.*, last Thursday), since they are useless when the chart is later reviewed.

Students (and interns) are often confused about whether to include information in the HPI or in the past medical history. It is a matter of preference. My personal approach is to list the past history in outline form *before* I describe the HPI, so as to "define the substrate" of the patient's problem.

Past medical and surgical history

See the section on Chart Review (page 18). Be sure to include an obstetric and menstrual history.

Medications

Include both current and recent medications, doses, recent changes in dose, and indications if they are not apparent. Accuracy in this section is crucial, since errors may lead to mis-administration of drugs. Medication lists are occasionally the only source of information about a patient's past medical history. Remember to use generic names. Finally, inquire about over-the-counter (OTC) medications, alternative therapies, and herbal or nutritional supplements.

> Examples:
> Amoxicillin 500mg tid, begun 9/1 for otitis.
>
> Verapamil-SR 240 bid, changed from qd 9/1.

You should know that attendings sometimes review medication lists to glean "objective" information when JMS presentations are confusing.

Developmental history

Include this section in pediatrics.

Family history

Psychiatric history

Screen for major depression

Include tobacco, alcohol, and other drug abuse including prior overdose.

Social history

Include an occupational history with attention to toxic exposures.

Note whether your adult patient (especially elderly or debilitated) lives alone or needs a caretaker. Begin your discharge planning now: determine if the home environment will be suitable for the patient's anticipated needs after discharge. Consider transportation obstacles including caretackers, distance, and cost.

Allergies & Hypersensitivities

See the comment in the "Orders" section on page 24.

Review of Systems

A good history of present illness contains a pertinent review of systems, so this section may not be necessary. Ask your attending.

Electronic health records enable careless box-checking. Avoid this.

Physical Exam

Here are some common JMS deficiencies in physical exams:

- **General appearance:** Whether or not the patient looks "ill" may be the most important part of the physical examination, and the most difficult part for the JMS to learn.

> Ask yourself "does this patient look sick?" every time you see one.

- **Vital signs** may be the second most important part of the physical examination. Measure vital signs **every** time you see your patients, especially when their condition suddenly changes. It may take you some time before you appreciate this simple advice.

> Know your patients' vital signs.

- **Genital and rectal exams:** You are not doing your patients a kindness by deferring examination of the groin, genitals, rectum, and skin.
- **Direct ophthalmoscopy** for examination of the fundus, as you probably already realize, takes lots of practice to master. Since funduscopic exams can be crucial during certain emergencies and can provide a wealth of information routinely, you should practice on **all** adult patients. After a few months you can become competent.

> Practice funduscopic exams with all patients. Check all routine admissions tests on the night of admission.

- **General approach:** Physical exams are tests just like any others you order; you should have specific questions in mind when you examine each organ system. For example, when you listen to lungs, ask yourself specific questions appropriate to the clinical situation, like "Are there signs of consolidation to suggest pneumonia? Are there signs of congestive heart failure?" Examining patients should not be the same as watching TV. Don't just lay that stethoscope to chest and stare glassy-eyed toward the hills, **attack** those lungs!

> Don't examine patients the same way you watch the yootubes; ask yourself specific questions in each part of the physical exam!

- **Laboratory tests:** You probably have been taught that the history and physical examination together suggest a diagnosis in the vast majority of illnesses. That is true, and usually laboratory tests are not helpful unless they answer a question raised by the history and physical. However, the population of adults sick enough to be admitted to the hospital (as opposed to outpatients) usually have many concurrent medical problems. In these people, a battery of laboratory tests are not only cost-effective, but quite powerful in identifying or excluding disease when combined with a good history and physical.

  As a corollary, important problems can be missed if you are not complete in your reporting of admission test results. Routine admission labs for adults on internal medicine include CBC/diff, chemistries, coagulation profile, ECG, chest radiograph, and urinalysis. Assume, for example, that as long as the urine has not been tested, it shows an abnormality.

  Be sure to include special bedside tests relevant to the patient's problem, like sputum gram stains for pneumonia, lumbar puncture for suspected meningitis, peripheral smear morphology for thrombocytopenia, *etc.* Indicate "tests pending" when necessary.

- **Problem list**

> *Lemme put this dogmatically:*
> The only way not to forget to address an important problem is systematically to list all problems in your admission note, and then to address each one in your assessment and plan.

  A problem list is just that: an enumeration of all the abnormalities unveiled by your diagnostic evaluation, grouped together whenever possible. Staring at a problem list can help you organize your thoughts about possible diagnoses, and about your diagnostic and therapeutic plan. For example, dyspnea, fatigue, orthopnea, paroxysmal nocturnal dyspnea, and edema might be grouped together under a single problem because together they suggest a limited differential diagnosis, most notably congestive heart failure; if you're not sure, list them separately.

- **Impression**

    Here is where you go to town. Write a concise but thoughtful essay about what you think is wrong with the patient. For each major element of the problem list, you should emphasize the differential diagnosis, and why this particular clinical scenario suggests certain elements of the differential more than it does others. You may want to speculate about the etiology and interrelation of problems. It usually helps to ask yourself, "Why does this patient have this problem? Why did the problem manifest now and not another time?" For example, congestive heart failure could be precipitated by a supervening infection or by medication noncompliance, among other things.

> Discuss the differential diagnosis of each problem and what precipitated the patient's decompensation.

- **Plans**

Once you have considered the differential diagnosis of every element on the problem list, you can formulate a course of action. For each problem you should describe your plans for further diagnostic evaluation, your plans for therapy, and your plans for patient education. The last is more important than you may at first think.

> How are you going to prove the diagnosis?
> How are you going to treat the illness?
> What are you going to tell the patient?

Copying-forward notes in electronic health records

One of the great crimes of American medicine is the tendency to recycle, electronically, electronic health records from the previous day or previous encounter. The result is a trash heap of verbose and unreliable blather.

Your patients deserve concise and unique medical notes created at each encounter. Moreover, completely-rewritten but concise notes help guide and organize your thinking.

> Do not copy-forward medical notes!

Internal Medicine Daily Progress Notes

Junior Medical Students write daily notes in the chart for each of the patients they follow. A note should summarize the new developments in a patient's hospital course, problems that remain active, plans to address those problems, and arrangements for anticipated discharge.

Daily notes force you to be compulsive. Ultimately, this benefits you because it helps you to stay on top of all your patient's problems, and answer almost any question your resident or attending might ask you about your patient.

Each note should address every element of the problem list from the previous day. Sitting down to write the note should amount to completing a checklist of everything that needed to be done that day. You need to talk to the patient to complete the subjective part of the note. You need to obtain vital signs and examine the patient thoroughly in order to record the physical exam. You need to find the results of tests in order to complete the labs section. And you need to sit back and review your patient's entire hospital course in order to reformulate an assessment and plan. Gaps in your daily care should become obvious when you sit down to write the note.

> Take better care of your patients than of your notes!

Remember that meticulous patient care is more important than meticulous note-writing. For the cynical: house staff and attendings do notice when you ignore your patients for the sake of your notes.

Most institutions recommend that medical students use a "SOAP" (Subjective, Objective, Assessment, and Plan) format for their daily progress notes.

- **Date/Time**

- **Subjective**

    Record patient reports of past problems, new problems, and the presence or absence of anticipated symptoms. For example, comment on appetite if the patient was anorectic, on postural lightheadedness if the patient had just been started on hypotensives.

- **Objective**

    This should include general appearance, vital signs, fluid inputs and outputs (I/Os), physical exam, labs, and current medications.

    Vital signs should include the highest temperature over past 24 hours. If a parameter has varied greatly, you should indicate the range (e.g., BP 120-160/70-100).

    I/O, including oral, parenteral, urine, and stool volumes. Weight, with a comment on trends.

    Physical exam

    Include chest and abdomen, with particular attention to active and anticipated problems. Emphasize changes from previous physical exams.

    Labs

    Include results of all new test results, circling abnormal values.

    Current medications

    Include medications as listed in the MTR, not the orders (see page 22). This list can be especially helpful in an emergency. Rewrite it frequently, even daily.

- **Assessment & Plan**

    Organize this by problem, writing a separate assessment and plan for each.

Sample progress note:
9/11/2020 Junior Medical Student Progress Note
Subjective: No fever overnight, productive cough persists, no new complaints. Orthopnea is resolved.

Objective:
VS: Tmax 37^4 - P80 - RR 14- BP 120/60
I/O: 1800 in/ 2400 out, net -600. Weight 68.7 kg, ↓ 0.8kg overnight, 2.2kg since admission.
PE:
Lungs: Rales without egophony at right posterior base, unchanged.
Cardiac: Regular rhythm, normal S1 + S2, no S3, (+) S4, no JVD, (+) hepatojugular reflux
Abdomen: Soft, nontender, active bowel sounds. Liver and spleen normal size.
Extr: Edema resolved.
Labs:
Na 135, K 3.6, Cl 110, HCO3 24, BUN 44, Cr 1.6.
Sputum culture: Pneumococcus sensitive to PCN.

Medications:
 Captopril 12.5 mg po tid.
 Furosemide 80 mg po qd.
 Cefuroxime 1.5mg IV q8°.

Assessment & Plan:
RLL Hospital-Acquired Pneumonia
Clinically improving, now afebrile on day 3/7 IV antibiotics. Culture reveals pneumococcus. Plan: Narrow antibiotic spectrum with penicillin IV

Congestive Heart Failure
Symptoms resolved with diuretics and afterload reduction. Tolerating higher dose of captopril. Prerenal azotemia despite persistent hepatojugular reflux probably reflects LV dysfunction despite excessive diuresis. Borderline hypokalemia also probably from diuretics. Plan: Lower diuretic dose, replete potassium more aggressively, advance captopril dose and check for postural hypotension, chest radiograph pending.
Discharge planning
No special needs anticipated.

Discharge Notes

At most hospitals, a complete summary of a patient's hospital course is dictated when the patient is discharged. The dictated summary may not actually be placed on the chart for many days or weeks. In the meantime, if a patient returns unexpectedly to the hospital or emergency department, a discharge note can serve as a temporary discharge summary.

Discharge notes contain virtually the same information as discharge orders, with the addition of a brief narrative. Here is a skeleton:

- Date/time.
- Diagnoses.
- Interventions (Write a single sentence describing therapy).
- Studies performed during the hospital stay.
- Test results outstanding at time of discharge (*e.g.*, interpretation of Holter monitor).
- Discharge medications.
- Follow-up arrangements.

Example:
5/14/2020 Junior Medical Student Discharge
Diagnosis: Congestive heart failure, E coli urinary tract

> infection
> Interventions: 7d IV antibiotics, successful diuresis.
> Studies: Renal ultrasound 5/7/2020, echocardiogram 5/10/2020
> Medications: Amoxicillin 500 mg po three times daily x 7d, Carvedilol 12.5mg twice daily, Lisinipril 20 mg daily
> Follow-Up: Dr. Hussein 5/21/2020 3:00 p.m.

Rather than write the same material twice, you can write "see discharge orders" for the list of medications and follow-up arrangements.

Surgery

Surgeons have an exceptional work ethic. In many ways, your surgery rotation may be the most challenging period of medical school. A few tips may make it easier.

First, always keep in mind that surgery residents are more tired and more over-worked than you are. They may not sympathize with your complaints about overwork or sleep deprivation.

Advance preparation is essential. Prepare for each surgical case before you scrub:

1. Review the disease being treated (*i.e.* pathophysiology, medical and surgical options, and the indications for surgical intervention.)

2. Master the relevant anatomy. For a laparoscopic cholecystectomy, know the arterial supply of the gallbladder, the pathways of the cystic, hepatic, and common bile ducts, and the relevant anatomy of the liver (the falciform ligament, the location of the IVC). Try to predict how you will be "pimped". You should expect to be asked about every layer of tissue between you and the target organ. When asked, "What am I cutting right now?" you need not answer "My pride." Don't be flustered if you're asked very difficult questions — surgeons like to ask you questions until you get one wrong.

> Study the disease and the anatomy the night before an operation!

Remember not to ask questions at inappropriate times during a procedure. That may be difficult for you to sort out at first. While the surgeons may appreciate an active learner, don't put the patient at risk because of your curiosity.

Responsibilities for students on a surgery service are difficult to define because surgical services are hierarchical yet team-oriented. One way to contribute significantly is to assume responsibility for the inpatient notes.

Surgery Pre-operative note

This note is intended to verify the patient is appropriately prepared for the operative procedure. Usually it is written the night, or visit, before scheduled surgery.

Procedure: Indicate what kind of surgery is planned (*e.g.,* exploratory laparotomy).

Labs: Include the results of a recent Chem-7, CBC, and PT/PTT. Make sure all of these tests are completed before surgery.

> A truly excellent JMS makes sure the blood bank has the blood available before surgery.

CXR (Chest X-Ray): For medicolegal reasons, surgeons often insist on an "official" reading from a radiologist.

ECG: An "official" reading from a cardiologist is often "necessary." Make sure you interpret the ECG yourself as well.

Urine: Note recent urinalysis or urine culture, *i.e.* that there is no unexpected infection before an elective procedure.

Consent: Assure that the patient understands and accepts the planned procedure, and that a consent form is "signed."

Diet: Make sure the patient is kept NPO (nothing by mouth) after midnight if general anesthesia is a possibility. Check the orders.

Diabetics typically need half their usual morning dose of insulin, and no oral hypoglycemic, if they are NPO before surgery.

Medications: Usually you will write "NPO except for medications." If perioperative antibiotics are planned, make sure they are ordered in advance.

The basic outline of a pre-op note follows, using the **SOAP** format:

> The preop note is like a "pre-flight" checklist. Make sure no item is "checked" unless it truly has been completed.

Example:

Date/Time: 3/23/2020 7:20 a.m.

Patient: P. Hagan

S: Patient pre-op for transcranial inguinal herniorrhaphy.

O: *Labs*: List all preoperative labs, specify if pending. Never leave blank spaces (add an addendum if necessary).

CXR: To detect subclinical cardiopulmonary abnormalities preop.

ECG: If obtained, results should be recorded.

Consent: ie, "Written informed consent."

A/P: Write pre-op orders (e.g. NPO, list bowel prep if applicable, IVF when NPO, etc.)

Surgery operative note
Residents will dictate a detailed operative note, but the transcribed report may take a long time to reach the chart. For the sake of the postoperative care team, a brief "Op note" is written in the chart, usually while the patient is still in the operating room. Remember, **"PPP SAFES FCDD"** for the standard headings: **Pre-operative diagnosis** (state the disease which necessitates the surgical procedure), **Post-operative diagnosis**, **Procedure** (list all procedures performed), Surgeons (the attending, residents and

medical students), **Anesthesia**, **Fluids** (the anesthesiologist has records of fluid balance and urine output), **Estimated blood loss** (EBL, get this information from the surgeon, nurses or anesthesiologist), **Specimens**, **Findings**, **Complications**, **Drains** (list them all), and **Disposition**.

> Example:
>
> 4/15/2020 10:20
>
> Pre-op Diagnosis: Colon Carcinoma.
>
> Post-op Diagnosis: same
>
> Procedure: Left hemicolectomy, time 3hrs 10 min.
>
> Surgeon: Curtis, MD
>
> Assistants: Slovo, MD, Calebresi, JMS
>
> Anesthesia: general endotracheal anesthesia (GETA).
>
> Fluids: Obtain all IV fluid totals from the anesthesiologist, as well as urine output.
>
> EBL (Estimated Blood Loss): 650 mL.
>
> Specimens: Mass, lymph nodes to pathology.
>
> Findings: A 3x4 cm mass in the descending colon with serosal involvement.
>
> Complications: ϕ.
>
> Drains: ϕ.
>
> Disposition: To recovery room in stable condition.

It is helpful to write a skeleton op note while you wait for the anesthesiologists to prepare the patient. Then you can complete the note immediately following the case.

Daily Surgery Progress Note

Surgery progress notes, in general, are much more concise than on an internal medicine service. In fact, resident notes may consist of two or three sentences. Student notes should be more complete, but remember that a two page progress note on a routine inpatient will look strange to the surgery residents. Just use the **SOAP** format:

> Example:
>
> 6/01/2020 9:35
>
> Patient:
>
> *S*: Indicate any new patient complaints. Does the patient have adequate pain relief? Is the patient now passing flatus or having bowel movements? How is the patient tolerating food? What kind of food is the patient eating? (e.g., nothing, clear liquids, soft, regular).
>
> *O*: <u>Maximum temperature</u> (T_{max}) and trend over past several days.
> <u>Current vital signs</u>.
> <u>Intake and Output</u>: volume of oral and intravenous fluids, volume of urine, stools, drains, and nasogastric output.
> <u>Weight and trend</u> over past several days.
> <u>Physical Exam</u>:
> - General appearance
> - Heart
> - Lungs
> - Abdomen
> - Comment on the wound/incision, e.g. "clean & dry," "serosanguinous drainage," "expressible pus," etc.
>
> <u>Lab results</u>: Look particularly for trends in white count, hematocrit, and electrolytes.
>
> *A/P*: These can be placed together under one heading.

> "Pt stable POD #2 s/p hemicolectomy
> - D/C NGT
> - Begin clear liquid diet, advance as bowel function returns
> - Leukocytosis and R basilar egophony: CXR
> - Will DC JP drain if < 50 mL drainage this shift
> - Likely discharge in 2 days to home with family"

Alternatively, a plan can be structured around systems, and this may be appropriate for the more complicated floor patients.

Quirks on surgical notes

Write out vital signs rather than writing "VSS" meaning vital signs stable. Actually writing them may compel you to check them.

- Be careful with the word "stable." Dead patients are "stable" too.
- Does the patient really need a Foley catheter? Often those are left in place through neglect.
- Do they still need that central vein catheter? When was that line last changed? Central and peripheral catheters left in place for more than several days are a risk for infection.
- Calcium, magnesium, and phosphorus are electrolytes, too. Check them if your patient has depended on you for nourishment.

Surgery Post-op note

A good surgeon's work only begins in the operating room. After every surgical procedure a "post-op check" is recorded in the chart. This is similar to a daily progress note with particular attention to a few important details:

Is the patient making enough urine? Because of postoperative fluid shifts, patients are often effectively volume-depleted (or overloaded). If urine output is less than 30 mL per hour, you may need to infuse fluids to prevent acute renal injury. Does the patient with tenuous cardiac function have pulmonary edema because of over-hydration? Evaluate the patient's volume status and call your intern now.

What are the respiratory rate, blood pressure, and heart rate? Don't trust the vital signs sheet. Measure them yourself if necessary.

> **Check vital signs!**

What is the temperature? A low-grade postoperative fever is often attributed to "atelectasis." Don't assume this too readily. Is the patient infected?

Check the wound/incision for excessive drainage or bleeding. Undress and examine the wound as appropriate in coordination with the nursing or physician staff.

> Do not allow an infected wound to hide behind dressings.
>
> Be respectful of staff who applied that dressing.

Don't hesitate to write the post-op note, generally two to six hours following surgery. Use the **SOAP** formula:

> Example:
>
> *Date/Time*: 5/25/2020 17:05
>
> *Patient*: S. Marvin
>
> *S*: Alert. Minimal nausea. No pain.
>
> *O*:
>
> *Vital Signs*: 37.8°C, HR 78 BP 124/68, s_aO_2 96%
>
> *Fluids*: NS 600 mL in, Urine 450 mL out, JP drain 20 mL out, net +130 mL
>
> *Physical Exam*: Lungs clear. Bowel sounds present. Dressing clean. (Always look at the dressing on the incision but never remove the dressing before 24 hours post-op unless specifically instructed.)
>
> *Labs*: Hb 12.4, Hct 48.3%

A/P: Pt stable s/p _____.

Volume status: Adequate urine output, vital signs appropriate.

Pain control: Adequate pain control with morphine PCA.

Diet: Ready for clear liquid, advance as tolerated.

Activity: Will move OOB to chair with assistance.

Obstetrics

Laboring patients tend to appreciate "coaching" from all members of the medical team, even from you!

The Labor Note

Be brief! Notes are recorded intermittently throughout labor by many members of the team. Try to write them whenever possible. Use **SOAP** format:

Guidelines:

Date/Time:
Patient:

S: Is the patient comfortable? Is analgesia adequate? Is she feeling contractions? How often? Other problems?

O: Record vital signs for mother, fetal heart tones, and vaginal exam.

Note the baseline heart rate and whether variability is adequate, and whether there are decelerations (early, late or variable). Early decelerations are usually caused by fetal head compression, late decelerations by placental insufficiency, and variable decelerations by cord compression.

For the vaginal exam, include details regarding cervical dilation and effacement as well as the "station" of the fetus in the mother's pelvis.

A: How is labor progressing? What stage?

P: Action taken. Note any internal monitors, anesthesia, or new medications. Also note if the patient is ready to push, or if an operative delivery is being considered. You may see your harried intern jot down the phrase "expectant management" when they are too busy with deliveries. A JMS should write more.

The Delivery Note

Organize delivery notes by the stages of labor.

Stage I: the onset of "true labor" to complete dilation of the cervix. True labor is progressive cervical effacement, dilation, or both, resulting from regular uterine contractions that occur at least every 5 minutes and last 30 to 60 seconds. When the woman has reached the end of stage I, she is said to "be complete" and is ready to push.

Stage II: complete cervical dilation to the birth of the baby.

Stage III: the birth of the baby to the delivery of the placenta.

Stage IV: delivery of the placenta to stabilization of the patient (usually about 6 hours post partum).

Guidelines:

Date/Time:

Patient:

Stage I: Reason for admission (i.e. 25 yo G1P0 at 40 weeks admitted at 0500 for S.R.O.M.) At what time did the patient progress to complete? Anesthesia? Pitocin used? If membranes ruptured following admission, note time and quality of fluid (clear or meconium-stained).

Stage II: How long did the patient push? Note any difficulty with the delivery and tools (forceps, vacuum) used to assist with delivery. Note the weight, sex, and Apgar scores (see below) of the baby. Note nuchal cord. Describe neonatal resuscitation efforts. Also include the cord blood gases.

Stage III: Describe the delivery of the placenta (spontaneous or manual) and describe the placenta briefly (i.e., intact, insertion of cord, number of vessels). Was uterine massage performed? Were medications (i.e., oxytocin) used to limit bleeding? Note estimated blood loss. Was an episiotomy performed? If there were lacerations, note the severity. A first-degree tear involves only the vaginal epithelium or perineal skin. A second-degree tear extends into the subepithelial tissues of the vagina, but does not involve the muscles of the perineal body. A third degree tear involves the anal sphincter and a fourth degree tear extends into the rectal mucosa. Describe the repair and anesthesia used. List physicians present.

Stage IV: Usually delivery notes are written before the completion of Stage IV. Include an explanation of any additional management or stabilization of your patient that occurred post-delivery. For example, include management of any peripartum hemorrhage.

Apgar Scores	0	1	2
Color	Blue/pale	Pink body/ blue extremities	Pink body & extremities
Heart rate	Absent	<100/minute	>100/minute
Reflex irritability	None	Grimace	Cough
Muscle tone	Limp	Some flexion	Full flexion
Respiratory effort	Absent	Weak cry	Strong cry

C-Section note
Use the "**PPP SAFES FCDD**" format as for other surgery op notes. In particular, under "findings" you will want to note the weight, sex, Apgar scores, and the position (vertex, breech) of the baby. Describe the appearance of the uterus, ovaries and fallopian tubes, and the placenta just as for a normal vaginal delivery note.

Post-partum notes:
Use the **SOAP** format. Be brief unless there are complications.

> Guidelines:
>
> Date/Time:
>
> Patient:
>
> **S**: How is the patient doing? Since the birth, is she walking, urinating without difficulty, and tolerating PO food? Is her lochia decreasing and is she having any pain?
>
> **O**: Vital signs, cumulative I/O's,
> Physical exam: Make note of the fundal height and the perineum. Is there lochia present at the perineum? If there was an episiotomy or a laceration repair, is the incision dry and without evidence of infection?
>
> **Assessment**: e.g., "Pt is a 25 yo G1P1 post partum day #1 following a NSVD, doing well."

Include contraception in the post-partum plan.

> **Plan**: Most patients will go home soon after delivery. You may wish to include: 1) follow up, 2) breast/bottle feeding and assistance to be provided (for breast-feeding), and 3) plans for contraception.

Pediatrics

Pediatrics history and physical exam

A carefully-written history and examination is important in pediatrics as for internal medicine. Parents provide most of the information about infants and small children.

Past Medical History (**PMH**) should include a birth history, vaccination status, developmental history, and social history.

> **The birth history** should include weeks of gestation, type of delivery, type of presentation if abnormal (ie, breech), and any complications from the perinatal period. Include maternal health during the pregnancy (i.e., mother tested positive for hepatitis B surface antigen, or mother used alcohol/drugs during pregnancy).
>
> **Vaccination status**. If all immunizations have been given on schedule, a simple "Vaccinations up-to-date" will suffice.
>
> **The developmental history** includes specific milestones, including:

	Motor	General	Social & Cognitive	Language and Speech
4 wks	Lifts head momentarily, intact reflexes	Follows object from midline to 90°, alerts to sounds	Early social smile	
8 wks	Lifts head 45 degrees		Social smile	Early cooing
3-4 mo	Lifts head 90 degrees	Lateralizes to sounds, Follows object from midline to 180°		Cooing
5-6 mo	Rolls front to back, voluntary grasp	Sits with propping	Smiles at image in mirror	Babbles with consonant sounds (ba, ma, ga)
7-10 mo	Finger-thumb	Sits without	Separation	Imitates sounds,

		apposition	support, localizes sounds in all directions	anxiety, object permanence	first words
12-15 mo		Builds tower of 2 blocks, learns to walk		Rolls ball to examiner	Understands one-step commands
15-18 mo		Builds tower of 4 blocks, improvement of walking		Can feed self with cup and spoon	Vocabulary of 10-50 words
24 mo		Runs without difficulty, beginning stairs		Parallel play	Vocabulary 50-75 wds, 2 word sentences

Social history: when considering the child's home, you should inquire about pets, since allergies and zoonoses are common.

Ask about pets!

Physical Exam: With children, it is especially important that you do a complete physical exam. Children should ALWAYS have their ears checked with an otoscope. In addition, their nares and oropharynx should always be examined for signs of edema or inflammation. Infections in these places are very common in kids.

Examine every ear you encounter on a child! Record height and weight on every physical exam. Identify trends by comparing with prior data.

Neonatal physical exams should include careful cardiac auscultation for congenital heart defects. Also perform Ortolani and Barlow maneuvers to identify congenital hip dislocation. With the thighs abducted, use your middle fingers to push the greater trochanters forward; a click with slippage of the femoral head signifies hip dislocation.

Outpatient Tips

Generally pediatrics consists primarily of outpatient health supervision and management of healthy children. Well-baby and well-child exams are mainly for screening and prevention. Many clinics will have a specific age-related checklist, *i.e.*smoke detectors, car-seats, seatbelts, environmental hazards, *etc.*

Neurology

Neurology is a wonderful challenge. A careful history can be exceptionally powerful. And of course, remain ever alert for confusion.

Neurology examination framework

Cognitive exam:

Level of consciousness: Alert-somnolent-stuporous-comatose). For patients with altered sensorium, especially after trauma, consider recording a **Glasgow Coma Scale**, a 15-point scale designed to predict mortality after traumatic head injury:

Score	Eye Opening	Best Motor	Best Verbal
1	None	No response	No response
2	To pain	Extension	Incomprehensible
3	To verbal	Flexion	Inappropriate
4	Spontaneous	Flexion withdrawal	Disoriented
5	---	Localizes to pain	Oriented
6	---	Obeys commands	---

When the patient is intubated use a "T" for best verbal response.

Orientation to person, place, and time.

Speech: Distinguish dysphasia from dysarthria.

Language, memory, cognition: For example, "Occasional paraphasic errors. Comprehends conversation but answers only "yes" or "no." Patient has difficulty embellishing answers to questions. Patient could identify fingers and a series of objects (pencil, pen, watch). Patient could not repeat numbers (5, 4, 3, 2, 1) or phrases. Patient seemed aware of political news, but could not easily express them (said 'Clinton . . . cigar . . . scandal'). Patient was unable to follow three-step commands." Is the patient able to perform calculations? Is the patient able to recall 3 objects after several minutes?

Cranial nerves:

Cranial Nerve	Simple test
I. Olfactory	Smell.
II. Optic	Visual fields and acuity.
III. Oculomotor	Pupil function and eye movements.
IV. Trochlear	Superior oblique muscle.
V. Trigeminal	Sensation of forehead, cheek, chin.
VI. Abducens	Lateral rectus muscle.
VII. Facial	Raise eyebrows, squint, smile and grimace, without asymmetry.
VIII. Vestibulo-cochlear	Hearing by rubbing fingers softly behind ear, tuning fork.
IX. Glosso-pharyngeal	Gag reflex.
X. Vagus	Symmetric palate and uvula movement.
XI. Accessory	Shrug and turn head against resistance.
XII. Hypoglossal	Asymmetry in protruded tongue.

Motor function

Examine function for each major muscle group: deltoids, biceps, triceps, wrist extensors, wrist flexors, dorsal interossei, hip flexors, knee extensors, knee flexors, plantar flexors, and dorsal flexors.

Tone: constant/lead pipe rigidity, cogwheel rigidity, increased spasticity, or prominent flaccidity of muscle groups.

Bulk: hypertrophy, atrophy, or normal

Strength: Make a chart of each major muscle group and grade strength:

0	Total paralysis
1	Flicker of contraction only
2	Movement if force of gravity is removed
3	Movement against gravity but not against added resistance
4	Movement can overcome partial degree of resistance
5	Full power

"**Pronator drift**", can detect subtle weakness. Ask the patient to raise both arms, palms up, to a ninety-degree angle, with their eyes closed. If there is "positive pronator drift'" the patient's arms will begin to pronate, or drift downward.

Coordination

Ask the patient to mimic **rapid alternating movements**, such as slapping the dorsal, then ventral surface of your hands on your knee in a rapid sequence. You can also ask them to touch their thumb to their index finger repeatedly, or to perform a **finger-to-nose** or **heel-to-shin** test. Include also a **Romberg** test. **Gait** encompasses strength, coordination, among other things. Have the patient stand and walk. Be sure to stand close to the patient in case they fall.

Sensory exam

This includes **light touch**, **temperature** (you can use the cool metal of your tuning fork), and **vibration**. If possible, try to describe the distribution of a sensory loss by the nerve distribution. You should also check and note **proprioception** or joint position sense. **Cortical or discriminative** sensation includes: **graphesthesia** by asking the patient, with eyes closed, to identify "writing" onto their hand or to identify an object placed into the hand. You can also test the patient's ability to **localize a pinprick** to a specific part of the body.

Reflexes

Draw a stick figure and note each reflex as :

Grade	Finding
0	Absent
1+	Hyporeflexic
2+	Normal
3+	Hyperreflexic

Include a **Babinski** test of dorsiflexion response to plantar stimulation.

Assessment

Based on your laborious history and physical examination, you should be attempt to localize the neurologic lesion and suspected pathology, **before** the results of an imaging study are available.

Psychiatry

Daily progress note should include:

General: Describe **appearance** including posture, grooming, and hygiene. Note **behavior**, including gestures and facial mannerisms. Finally, note the patient's **affect** or **demeanor**. Is the patient hostile or pleasant? Cooperative or avoidant? Does the patient seem mentally "slow"?

State of consciousness: Is the patient alert, drowsy, stuporous, or obtunded?

Attention and concentration: Observe for hyperalertness or hyperacusis. Notice whether the patient is preoccupied by other thoughts. Does the patient seem easily distracted by other stimuli in the environment?

Ask the patient to perform "digit recall". Simply speak a series of numbers and ask the patient to repeat them back to you. Start with a set of three numbers and increase the amount of digits to recall as the patient succeeds. Keep in mind that a normal maximum is seven numbers. The patient's ability to concentrate can be evaluated by asking them to spell a simple word, such as "CAT" or "WORLD" backwards.

Speech: Comment on the patient's quality of speech. Is it loud, soft, fast, slow, pressured (pushed to speak quickly), *etc*? Does the patient articulate clearly? Listen for words that you don't recognize or that are chosen inappropriately.

Orientation: Check for orientation to person, place, time, and situation (Does the patient realize why they are in your care?). Suitable questions include: What is today's date, the day of the week, the month, the season, or the year? Where are we now? What is your full name? Where were you born? What is your spouse's name? Remember that the first orientations to be lost are to situation and to time.

Mood and affect: Don't confuse these two terms! Mood is a sustained emotional state, such as a state of depression, euphoria, or anxiousness. Affect is the patient's current emotional state. For example, to the examiner, a patient's affect may appear blunted, flat, or inappropriate.

Thought: Includes both **form and content of thought**. Form of thought pertains to the way in which patients string thoughts together. Does one thought follow another logically? Does the patient display circumstantial reasoning (including many irrelevant details, taking forever to make a point)? Does the patient exhibit flight of ideas (rapidly jumping from one thought to another with no connection) or perseveration (needless repetition of the same thought or phrase)? Abnormalities in form of thought are common in schizophrenia and schizoaffective disorders.

The patient may have **delusions** or fixed, false beliefs not related to the patient's culture or background. For example, "I am being followed constantly by the FBI, and I know they are here looking for me in the hospital." **Hallucinations** are false sensory perceptions, such as hearing voices that are not present, or seeing objects that do not exist. **Illusions** are an abnormal interpretation of existing stimuli; for example, "I know that the lamp in the corner of my room is a listening device for the aliens that are chasing me." Always note any thoughts of **suicide** or **homicide**.

Evaluate capacity for **abstract** thinking. Ask for the meaning of a simple proverb, such as "What does it mean when I say people in glass houses shouldn't throw stones?" The response, "The phrase means you shouldn't throw stones against glass because it can break." is an example of "concrete thinking."

Judgment demonstrates capacity for independent functioning. Ask, for example, "What would you do if you found a stamped, addressed letter on the ground?"

Memory: Test immediate, recent, and remote memory. Have the patient remember three words or digits (immediate memory), and then at the end of the interview have the patient recall them (recent memory). Remote memory involves recall of events that occurred more than 24 hours in the past. You can ask about any significant historical event in the past year, to name the previous four presidents, to describe how the patient celebrated her last birthday, *etc*.

Intellectual Function: Estimate this from the general tone and content of the interview, as well as by the patient's general scope of knowledge. Easy questions to ask include: "How many dimes are there in $1.20?; How much change do I get back if I buy a soda for $1.30 and I give the cashier $2.00?; Why do birds fly south in the winter?; and What does the heart do?"

Procedures

You should jump at every opportunity to do procedures, from phlebotomy to arthrocentesis to central line placement. Supervised practice is important, because in a few years a patient's life may depend on your deft performance of a procedure as simple as phlebotomy or intravenous catheter placement; immediate help won't always be available. Phlebotomy and IV placement are also good ways to make yourself useful to the team during early clerkships.

Know that junior house officers usually have priority learning how to do special procedures, especially early in the year. Ultimately that is better for patient care, but frustrating for a JMS.

Preparing for any procedure

- Read about procedures before doing them. Even the first time, when you have a resident by your side, you should know in advance exactly what you are about to do and why. You should know the likely complications and how you will respond when they happen.

- Prepare all supplies in advance, including those you will need in case your initial attempt fails. For example, take extra syringes and needles for phlebotomy, so that you don't have to find extras and start all over in case you miss.

- Gather correct materials for submitting specimens to the laboratory, including patient identification labels and requisitions. Make sure the laboratory is prepared to accept the specimen (for example, cytology specimens on weekends).

- Prepare disposable dropcloths (*e.g.,* Chux) so you don't create any unnecessary mess. Remember to clean up after you are finished; other staff resent picking up after house officers and students.

- Make sure both you and the patient are comfortably positioned.
- The "field" should be well illuminated.

- You should be protected appropriately against injury. In the days of the giants, getting covered with blood and stool was a matter of pride. Unfortunately, such body substance exposure represents a serious risk, by exposing you to blood-borne infection (See the section on Universal body substance isolation on the following page)
- Make sure your hands are clean, or that you are sterile-scrubbed, as appropriate.
- Make sure the patient understands and consents to the procedure.

Act swiftly and assuredly.

Style can be everything in performing a procedure. Act with "humble confidence." It reassures the patient and makes success more likely. Remember that the hesitant style of overly cautious Junior Medical Students can guarantee failure. For example, it hurts to advance a needle too slowly/cautiously during phlebotomy. And arteries invariably roll out of the way when you advance a needle too slowly obtaining an arterial blood gas.

Universal body substance isolation

Here are modified CDC guidelines for minimizing your risk of acquiring HIV and hepatitis B virus in the health-care setting:

Treat all patients as if they have a blood-borne infection.

Wash hands before and after all patient contact, and after removing gloves. Wash them immediately if you contaminate your skin with blood or other body fluids.

Wear gloves when it is likely that you will soil your hands with blood or body fluids.

Wear protective eyegear if splattering with blood or body fluids is possible, which is every procedure.

Be very careful with contaminated needles and other disposable sharp objects. When you have a contaminated sharp object in your hand, your top priority should be to place that object safely into a puncture-resistant container located in every patient room.

Do not recap or bend the needle. Do not lay the sharp object down on a bed, **ever**. Do not overfill containers with sharps.

Treat contaminated sharps as deadly weapons. Note that bags and masks for ventilating patients should readily be available in areas where resuscitation procedures are likely.

Gowns are not mandatory unless it is likely you will soil exposed skin or clothing, or unless you plan a durable implant such as a central venous line.

If have open lesions, dermatitis, *etc.*, you should refrain from direct patient care and from directly handling contaminated equipment, and you should contact a physician.

Introduction to Phlebotomy & IV Placement

This is the bread and butter procedure for a JMS or a house officer. Drawing blood and starting IV's requires skill and practice. It should not be seen as demeaning "scut work."

Finding and filling a vein
Making a vein distend is the most important part of phlebotomy and IV placement. Veins are flabby and difficult to cannulate when empty, but easy to pierce when filled with blood.

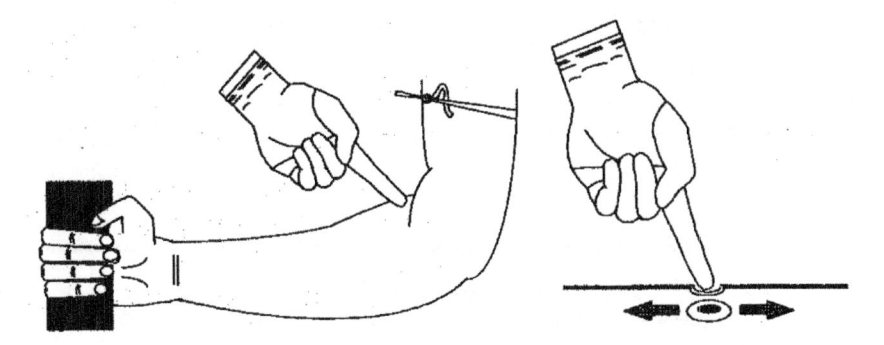

Get to know the characteristic feel of veins under skin: soft and particularly distensible along the middle. Practice feeling your own arm veins all the time, when they are empty and when they are full, when you are warm and when you are cold. See how they roll aside when you press them eccentrically.

Learn how to distinguish veins from tendons in your antecubital fossa and the dorsum of your hand. Milk the blood in a vein distally (retrograde) and see how valves distend. Know that it is challenging and undesirable to pass an IV catheter through a venous valve.

There are several ways to make arm veins fill, even if you can't see them:

- Tourniquets are most common. Make sure that the arm is held lower than the heart before you apply the tourniquet. Make sure the tourniquet is neither too tight (obliterating arterial inflow) nor too loose (not obstructing venous outflow). A most excellent trick is to use a blood pressure cuff as a tourniquet. Pump the cuff to a pressure less than systolic but more than about 40mm Hg. If veins exist, they will appear within two minutes. This technique is especially helpful for placing IV catheters in the very old; it usually is unnecessary for a routine blood draw.

- Ask the patient to pump the wrist with the tourniquet in place. Note that this may distort certain blood tests.

- Apply a warm compress (a towel or diaper with hot, not scalding, water) for a few minutes. This works especially in the very young and the very old.

- Try slapping the area of interest briskly for ten or twenty seconds. (Note: the "slapping" should be quick and light!).

Never apply a tourniquet for more than five or ten minutes. It hurts, and metabolic derangements will alter chemistry results (especially potassium, bicarbonate, and lactate). You can always reapply the tourniquet after a few minutes and try again.

Don't forget to remove tourniquets!

Always remember to remove the tourniquet! This is a common JMS blunder. It can explain why IV fluids won't flow into a new and functioning catheter. It can also cause an ischemic extremity.

Selecting a vein for phlebotomy
It is usually easiest to select a vein once all the veins are distended. Use the techniques described above before making your selection. Common sites for phlebotomy include:

- The antecubital fossa (the opposite side of the elbow).

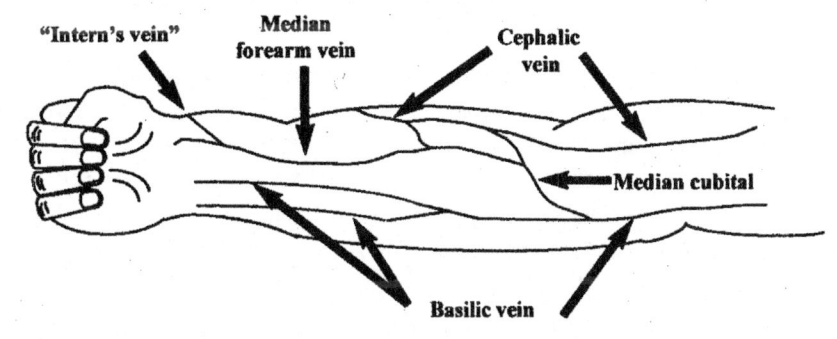

Labeled diagram of arm veins: "Intern's vein", Median forearm vein, Cephalic vein, Median cubital, Basilic vein.

- The veins on the dorsum of the hand, especially at a point where two veins join, thereby "tethering" the site against an advancing needle.
- Veins on the lateral thenar eminence.
- The cephalic vein on the wrist and on the lateral aspect of the forearm. Save this for IV's if you can.
- The basilic vein on the medial aspect of the forearm.

Choice of needles
Small needles cannulate blood vessels more easily and hurt less; however they may damage or hemolyze red cells. Small IV catheters may not pass fluids quickly enough for patients requiring rapid fluid resuscitation and may damage transfused blood. On the other hand, large needles hurt, damage blood vessels, and increase the likelihood of failed phlebotomy or IV placement. Note that thicker IV catheters are also usually longer.

82...Procedures — Truly Excellent Junior Medical Student

> Needles for adults:
> IV's: 18G or 20G.
> Phlebotomy: 23G or larger.
> Arterial blood: 25G.

Needle diameter is specified as gauge, with larger numbers representing narrower needles. When drawing blood, 23G needles won't hemolyze the specimen if the blood is drawn slowly. For arterial blood gas measurements, a 25G needle is used to minimize arterial trauma, but the blood may hemolyze. 18G IV catheters, which are large enough to hurt, are usually adequate for most patients, except hemorrhaging patients who may require several 16G or even 14G catheters.

Inexperienced JMSs should learn using 20G IV catheters and then progress. For elderly or pediatric patients, a 22G IV may be adequate.

Three types of equipment are commonly used for phlebotomy: syringe and butterfly, syringe and straight needle, or vacutainer.

> Butterfly needles are easiest.

Butterfly needles have butterfly-shaped plastic handles and flexible plastic tubing which can be connected to a syringe. Butterflies are especially maneuverable and easy to use. With this setup, you draw blood into a syringe and then transfer it to tubes afterwards. Since the tubing isolates the needle from the syringe, it is difficult to jar the needle out of a cannulated vessel in the middle of drawing blood. The clear tubing permits you to see the "flash" of blood when you hit the vessel.

If you can't find a butterfly needle, you can just attach a **straight needle** to a syringe. This works just fine in young people who have large veins. However, a little jerk of the hand may destroy a fragile vein and your phlebotomy will fail.

Vacutainers are needles sharp at both ends held in a rigid plastic device. You cannulate a blood vessel and then stick a vacuum blood tube onto the other end until it fills. You can fill as many tubes this way as you want, if you have a steady hand. Vacutainers have the same disadvantages as syringes with straight needles, except you can't see the "flash" when you cannulate the vessel. Vacutainers aren't good for veins on the dorsum of the hand, which tend to collapse when vacuum is applied. Professional phlebotomists use vacutainers for speed. Vacutainers are cool, but hard to use. Start with something easier.

Tubes

Blood is submitted to the laboratory in several different test tubes. Specimens are submitted to the laboratories in a similar way at most institutions:

- **Red-top** or **red-gold** or **"tiger-top"** tubes are for tests on serum, like chemistries (electrolytes, glucose, liver enzymes, bilirubin, protein & albumin, lipids, *etc.*), serologies and antigens (*e.g.*, type & cross for transfusion, hepatitis B antibodies and antigens, HIV ELISA and Western blot), *etc.* Serum is blood devoid of cells and clotting factors, so there are no anticoagulants in red-tops. In fact, the blood must clot before the serum is removed. **Red-gray**-top tubes are a variant of red-tops which contain a yellow plug. When these tubes are spun in a centrifuge, the plug interposes between the serum and cells, making serum removal easier. For most purposes, these tubes are interchangeable.

Red tops are for serum chemistries.

- **Lavender-top** tubes are for tests on blood cells, like complete blood count, leukocyte differential, peripheral smears, erythrocyte sedimentation rates, *etc.* Obviously clotting would interfere with these tests, so there is a fixed volume of EDTA solution. If you add only a small volume of blood to a lavender-top, it will be diluted by the liquid anticoagulant and the hematocrit will artifactually be low.

Lavender tops are for blood counts, ESR.

- **Blue-top** tubes are for clotting measurements, especially prothrombin time (PT) and partial thromboplastin time (PTT). These tubes contain a measured amount of the calcium-chelator sodium citrate; to measure clotting parameters, calcium is later added. *If you underfill or overfill a blue-top tube, the PT and PTT will be inaccurate.*

> Blue tops are for PT & PTT.

- **Green-top** tubes are for STAT processing of chemistries at most hospitals. They contain lithium heparin and yield plasma not serum; for some reason automated chemistries can be performed much faster on plasma.

> Green tops are for STAT chemistries.

- **Grey-top** tubes are for testing glucose, blood alcorhol, or lactic acid. They contina sodium fluoride or sodium oxalate to prevent glycolysis or clotting, respectively. This allows delayed specimen testing.

Tubes come in standard (5-10mL) and small (1.5-2mL) sizes. Most routine tests can be performed on small volumes of blood, so collect the blood in small tubes wherever possible. Obviously it is easier and faster to collect less blood than more. Also, repeated phlebotomy sometimes causes frank anemia in patients during a lengthy hospital stay.

> Use small-volume tubes when possible.

Blood tubes should be filled with care. All contain a vacuum and will fill automatically once you insert the needle/syringe through the rubber stopper. *Never apply additional pressure* on a syringe to fill a tube faster; this will hemolyze red cells, altering electrolyte measurements and CBC morphology. As mentioned above, purple and especially blue-top tubes are designed to hold a specific quantity of blood; overfilling or underfilling these tubes will result in inaccurate test results.

> Don't fill blood stoppered tubes with pressure.

Performing venipuncture

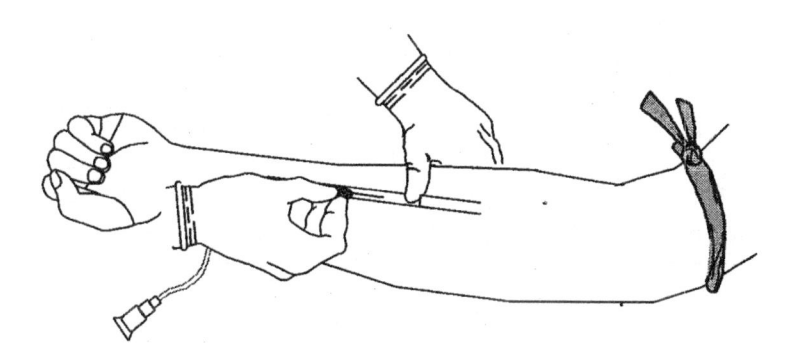

Supplies for venipuncture

- Needle apparatus described above, with extra needles in case of failure
- Tubes for submitting blood specimens (see page 88)
- Tourniquet or cuff
- 4x4" cotton gauze pads
- Alcohol swabs
- Latex gloves

Drawing the blood

Calculate how much blood you need to draw. Ask your house officer for help.

Get comfortable. Make sure the patient is comfortable too.

Apply a cuff or a tourniquet. Tuck a free end of the tourniquet underneath the skin in such a way that a short tug will release it.

Select a vein (see page 93). **Palpate** the venous site you have chosen. Anticipate how it will roll.

Alcohol stings when you draw blood.

Swab the site with alcohol. Know that alcohol is not particularly bactericidal. Remove **gauze** pads from wrapper. Wait for the alcohol to dry or wipe it dry with sterile gauze.

> Put on gloves!

Quickly and deftly drive the needle into the vein. You can only learn by practice. Just remember not to be overly hesitant as you insert the needle. Although you may not recognize it the first dozen times, you can feel a characteristic "pop" when you insert a needle into a vein. A butterfly needle provides a visual cue when you are in the right place: a drop of blood runs into the clear tubing.

Veins that are fragile or that "roll" away from needles are sometimes best punctured in two stages: (1) puncture the skin aiming away from the vein, and (2) puncture the vein from within the subcutaneous tissue.

If you miss the vein completely, withdraw the needle until it is just underneath the skin, re-aim, and make another attempt.

If you miss but damage a vein, you may see blood spilling out of the vein into the subcutaneous space. Quickly remove the tourniquet, remove the needle, and **compress** the site with a gauze pad. Elevating the arm above the heart may prevent a hematoma.

Withdraw as much blood as you need.

Remove the tourniquet while leaving the needle in place. Otherwise blood will pour out of the vein and cause a hematoma and a mess.

Grab the gauze pad, smoothly withdraw the needle, and compress the venipuncture site

Compress the venipuncture site for 3-4 minutes until it doesn't bleed. You can ask the patient to do this for you. At the very least, you want to preserve this site for future phlebotomy, so take good care of it. It is very bad form not to obtain adequate hemostasis.

Recapping needles is dangerous! Without recapping, discard the needles and syringes in the special boxes provided in every room for blood-contaminated sharp objects.

Clean up after yourself.

Submit your blood specimens to the laboratory.

Placing IV's

Indications for placement of IV's
- Medications
- Fluids
- Parenteral alimentation
- Hemodynamic instability

Some patients may suddenly deteriorate, requiring IV access for rapid fluid and medication infusion. This includes patients undergoing surgery, patients with a recent GI hemorrhage, and patients on cardiac monitors. These patients should have an IV "just in case."

Common complications of IV access
- Pain and discomfort.
- Local infection, including suppurative phlebitis and cellulitis.
- Systemic infection, including sepsis, infective endocarditis, infection of prosthesis (artificial joints and valves, vascular grafts).
- Thrombosis and thromboembolism, especially in lower extremity IV's.
- Destruction of venous sites for future phlebotomy and IV access.

Considerations in placing IV catheters
- **Distal location**

    When IV's fail, the vein often becomes inflamed or thrombosed. More proximal segments of the same vein may remain patent (because of collaterals), while distal segments may occlude. For this reason it is best to preserve proximal sites by placing IV's as distally as possible.

- **Vulnerability**

    Sometimes IV's must be placed in joint creases (antecubital fossa, proximal wrist). To guard the IV, the joint usually must be immobilized with a stiff arm board.

- **Size**

    See "choice of needles" on page 86.

- **Comfort**

    IV's should be put in non-dominant arms when possible. Avoid sites that require joint immobilization.

- **Ongoing need, urgency of replacement**

    Patients who have IV's one day may not need them the next. Because of the discomfort and risk of infection, reevaluate the need for IV catheters every day. Make sure you let the nurses or cross-covering interns know that if the IV falls out, it needn't be replaced immediately.

- **Age of catheter**

    The longer a given IV is left in place, the more likely it will get infected. At some hospitals, IV's are replaced routinely after 3-4 days. When a patient develops a fever in the hospital, one of the first management steps is to remove and culture all IV catheters.

Selecting a vein for an IV

These are the easiest and most comfortable sites to place IV's:

- Cephalic vein.
- Dorsal hand veins.
- "Intern's" vein, in the anatomic "snuff box".
- Basilic vein.
- Volar forearm veins are difficult.

When you have exhausted the above possibilities, you can try some of the following less desirable sites:

- Antecubital fossa: less desirable because it is in a joint crease.
- External jugular: a straightforward cannulation site, frightening only because it is in the neck. Not for the inexperienced.
- Deep brachial vein: This vein runs just medial to the brachial artery, on the posteromedial aspect of the biceps. Since the vein is so deep, this is a "blind stick:" you aim for a point just medial to the pulsating brachial artery, which you can feel but not see. **Don't puncture the brachial artery,** since the forearm may not have good collateral arteries. Proximal arm sites like these are best accessed under ultrasound guidance.

Where not to place an IV catheter:
- Through an area of compromised skin, like a burn or infection.
- Ipsilateral to a mastectomy or axillary lymph node dissection, since these predispose to systemic infection.
- On a lower extremity, especially in a patient with vascular disease like diabetes mellitus. These predispose to phlebitis, cellulitis, and thromboembolic complications.
- Through a renal dialysis graft or fistula or in the days before a graft or fistula is placed in the same arm.
- Through the saphenous vein of a patient who may soon require coronary artery bypass grafting.

Supplies for IV placement
- IV catheters. At most institutions, flexible latex catheters are available with removable steel needles inside of them (*e.g.,* Angiocath brand). In some catheters, the needles themselves are hollow, so that you can draw blood through the catheter when you first place it.
- Tourniquet or cuff.
- Blood-drawing syringe, tubes, and needles if you plan to draw blood from the IV.

90...Procedures *Truly Excellent Junior Medical Student*

- Saline lock (aka HepLock). This is a rubber-capped tube that you can attach to the end of the IV catheter. Medications or fluids can be directly injected into the IV through the rubber cap. With a HepLock in place, a patient can be freed from IV tubing while the IV site is kept intact.
- DO NOT mistake heparin (1,000 unit/mL) for HepLock flush (1 unit heparin/mL). HepLock flush. This is a very dilute heparin solution. Draw the flush into a 5mL syringe and leave the needle on the syringe. Most centers now use normal saline so as not to sensitize patients to heparin.
- A roll of 1"-wide clear-plastic surgical tape.
- Chux, disposable diaper-like absorbent dropcloths.
- 4x4" gauze pads.
- Povidone-iodine or chlorhexidine pads or swabs.
- Alcohol pads.

> Bring along at least one extra catheter, in case you miss during your first attempt.

Inserting the IV
Now it's time to insert the IV. Everybody does this differently, and everybody does it badly at first. Here is my way:

Setup
Select a vein (see above).

Prepare the Heplock. Draw 3-5mL "Heplock flush" into a 5mL syringe with a needle. Insert the needle into the rubber end of the Heplock and flush it to expel the air. Leave the needle/syringe in the Heplock and place the apparatus within easy reach.

Prepare strips of tape. You will need a 6" x 1/2" piece for a "chevron" and a few wider 6" strips to secure the HepLock and catheter. Stick these to the side of the bedrails for easy reach.

Apply tourniquet/cuff and palpate the site to get comfortable with the vein. Anticipate how the vein will roll as you insert the IV. Make sure there are no valves proximal to the insertion site for the length of the IV catheter.

Put "chux" underneath the arm.

Prepare a sterile field: paint the insertion site with povidone-iodine swabs three times and then swab the inside with alcohol, as described in "blood cultures section (page 99).

Wash and glove your hands, protect your eyes.

1. Loosen the latex catheter from the steel needle, so that they will separate easily later.

Cannulate

Cannulate in two steps. It is easier to puncture but not damage a vein when the needle is already underneath the skin.

1. Tether the vein by pulling the skin distal to the insertion site.
2. Decisively pierce the skin with the needle, bevel-up, aiming proximally, and making an angle of about 30° with the skin. Aim to the side of the vein; you will puncture that afterwards.

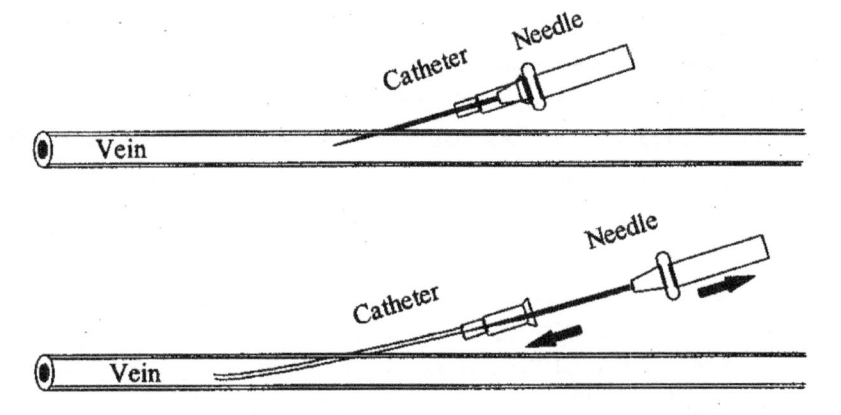

3. Once you have penetrated the skin, angle the catheter so it is more parallel to the skin.
4. In a second decisive thrust, pierce the vein itself. Once you are inside, you will see a "flash" of blood inside the IV catheter. Advance the needle only a couple of millimeters further; any more and you may damage the vein; any less and the vein may rupture when you try to slide the catheter

inside. Avoid through-and-through puncture through both front and back walls.

> With experience you will feel a characteristic "pop" when the catheter enters the vein.

5. If you miss but do not cause a hematoma, you may want to leave the "ectopic" angiocath in place for temporary hemostasis while you place another IV in the same arm. Holding the needle in place, slide the latex catheter forward into the vein. You should see blood enter the space between the needle and the catheter. Advance until the nub almost abuts the skin.
6. Remove the tourniquet.

Secure and clean-up
1. Grab the HepLock apparatus in one hand, and the nub of the catheter in the other. Quickly remove the needle from the IV and replace it with the HepLock. Don't bump the IV or you may damage the vein.

> Make sure the tourniquet is removed.

2. Flush the catheter with the HepLock flush you prepared. If the IV flushes without resistance, you have a good IV. Otherwise, you may see the IV site infiltrate with fluid.
3. Without disturbing the IV, make a "chevron." Take the long & narrow piece of tape and place it, adhesive side up, behind the IV nub. Cross the free ends of tape and attach to skin on opposite sides.
4. Remove the povidone-iodine stain and blood with alcohol pads.
5. Secure the IV with additional clear plastic tape.
6. Clean up your mess. Let a nurse know that a HepLock is in place. Document as required.

Blood Culture

An essential component of the infamous "fever workup" is phlebotomy for blood culture. It is said that cultures have the greatest yield when they are obtained just as the temperature begins to rise, or while the patient has frank rigors.

A common mistake on some services is to start empirical antibiotics before blood cultures are obtained. Circulating antimicrobials may sterilize blood culture, and the lack of a bacteriological diagnosis can be dangerous for the patient. As the JMS you can make sure this doesn't happen.

> Obtain blood cultures before giving antimicrobials.

Most hospitals culture blood in special culture medium bottles which are processed by machine. In general, blood specimens are divided and submitted in two bottles, one for aerobic organisms and one for anaerobic organisms. For a new fever, you usually obtain two "sets" each of two bottles, drawn from different sites and fifteen minutes apart. If the patient has a central line, obtain one of the specimens from that line and label the requisition as such. In circumstances when you suspect disseminated mycobacterial disease, submit a third mycobacterial bottle (red) for each "set."

It is essential to use good aseptic technique when obtaining blood for culture, since the culture bottles will grow contaminants as well as pathogens. If you accidentally contaminate a bottle with skin organisms, your patient's management can become very confusing and difficult. Growing a skin organism, like coagulase-negative staphylococci, from only one of two culture bottles is often a clue that the organism is a contaminant. On the other hand, if the patient has a prosthetic heart valve and grows coagulase-negative staphylococci from only one bottle, that patient still likely will be committed to weeks of potentially toxic intravenous antimicrobials.

> Good aseptic technique is crucial for blood culture.

Supplies for blood culture
- Blood-drawing apparatus, *e.g.*, butterfly and syringe, tourniquet, gloves, 4x4" cotton gauze, chux, and extras as needed.
- An additional sterile needle (usually 18G).
- Blood culture bottles, at least two.
- Three sets of povidone-iodine (Betadine brand) swabs or pads.
- One alcohol pad for the patient, and one more for each blood culture bottle.

Phlebotomy for blood culture
1. Remove the caps from the blood culture bottles without touching the tops. Remove the bottle tops and disinfect the latex tops with alcohol pads.
2. Apply the tourniquet and select a vein as for any phlebotomy. Palpate the vein well.
3. Swab the venous site with povidone-iodine or chlorhexidine disinfectant in a spiral fashion, from the inside outwards. In this way the phlebotomy site will be in the center of a sterile circle of disinfectant. Be sure not to move the swab from a "contaminated" area of skin to a "sterile" area already swabbed. Repeat this for a total of three sterile swabs. Wait for the disinfectant to dry.

> Swab from the "sterile" to the "contaminated" parts of the field.

4. Repeat the sterile "prep" above if you accidentally contaminate the sterile field. Do not touch the site with your finger, unless you are wearing sterile gloves.
5. Draw 6-10mL of blood from the venous site you identified earlier. Do not touch the site with your contaminated finger. At least do not touch the area of skin through which the needle is passing.

6. Remove the tourniquet, withdraw the needle, remove it from the syringe without contaminating it, and discard the (uncapped) needle immediately into the appropriate container.
7. Apply the gauze with pressure to the phlebotomy site.
8. Without contaminating the needle or the specimen, transfer 3-5mL of blood into each blood culture bottle.
9. Discard the syringe and (uncapped) needle into the appropriate container.
10. Clean up. This includes washing away blood and colorant.
11. Submit your specimens to the laboratory. Do not refrigerate blood culture bottles.

Arterial Blood Gas

Obtaining blood for arterial blood gas (ABG) determination is different in many respects. It is more painful. It is done more by palpation than visualization. Specimens must be obtained in heparinized syringes and must be placed immediately on ice.

Blood is usually obtained from the radial artery. If that is not possible, consult your house officer before performing femoral or brachial artery puncture.

Arterial puncture is often much easier than phlebotomy. However, because of the risk of complications, it is generally inappropriate to perform arterial blood sampling to avoid difficult venipuncture.

Indications for arterial blood gas
- To confirm clinical suspicion of hypoxia, carbon dioxide retention, acid-base abnormality, methemoglobinemia, carbon monoxide poisoning.
- To assure adequate oxygenation or ventilation in patients receiving supplemental oxygen or mechanical ventilation.

Non-invasive pulse-oximetry can substitute for repeated ABGs for oxygenation.

Complications
- Arterial thrombosis and ischemic extremity
- Arterial trauma or aneurysm
- Hematoma
- Infection

Supplies for ABG
- Ready-heparinized 1-3mL syringe. Nowadays all the supplies you need are available in kits, but if you can't find one, you can heparinize your own syringes: Draw some heparin solution (not HepLock flush) into the syringe, and draw the plunger up and down a few times, with the syringe upside down, to coat the sides with heparin. Expel almost all of the heparin immediately before obtaining the blood specimen.
- 25G needle for radial puncture, or 1.5" 20G needle for femoral puncture.
- 4x4" gauze bandage.
- Small towel for leverage.
- Small bag full of ice.
- Cap for submitting the syringe without a needle.

Radial artery puncture for arterial blood gas

Before radial artery puncture, you would traditionally perform the **Allen test** to make sure the hand will be perfused in case you thrombose the radial artery. Using both hands, occlude the radial and ulnar arteries, and ask the patient to pump and relax a fist several times. Now keep pressure on the radial site while letting go of the ulnar site. Watch how color returns to the hand. Repeat while releasing the radial site only. Radial artery puncture is contraindicated if it takes longer for color to return with the ulnar occluded than with the radial occluded.

Prepare for radial puncture:

1. Get comfortable.
2. Have the patient rest and supinate the forearm on side of the bed or chair. Roll up the small towel and put it under the dorsal surface of the wrist. This forces the patient to dorsiflex the wrist, which helps prevent the radial artery from rolling away from the needle. No tourniquet is necessary.

> **Beware of superficial veins overlying the artery. Remember the radial artery can be very superficial.**

3. Assuming you are right-handed, palpate the radial artery with your left hand just proximal to the wrist. Feel the artery along a 1cm stretch and picture in your mind exactly where the artery runs. Imagine the lateral boundaries of the artery as well. Some people palpate the artery with two fingers, with the intention of inserting the needle between their fingers.
4. Clean the skin with an alcohol swab.
5. Prepare the 4x4" gauze pad.
6. "Unfreeze" the piston of the syringe by moving it slightly.
7. Explain to the patient that this will likely hurt more than venipuncture.
8. Aim the needle at the artery, bevel up, making a 45°angle with the skin, pointing proximally.
9. Thrust the needle through the skin and through the posterior wall of the artery in one smooth motion.

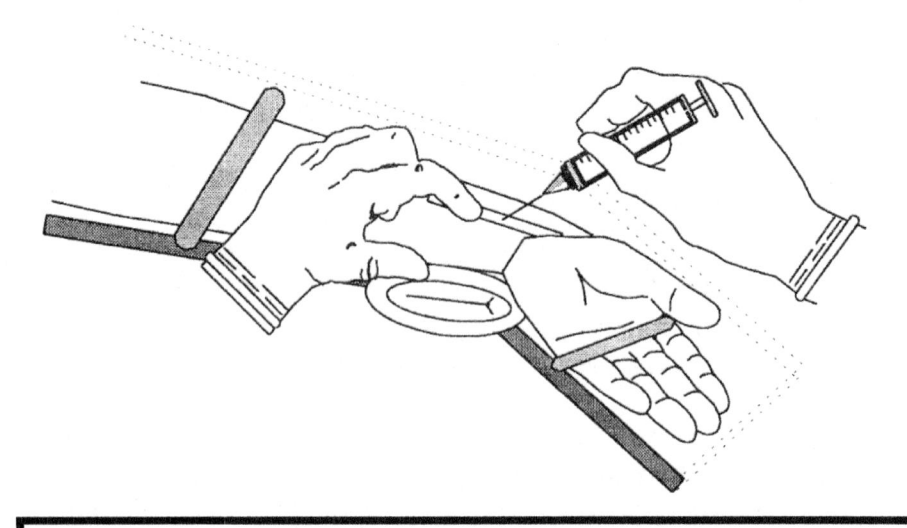

> Arterial pulsations confirm an arterial over venous entry.

10. Slowly withdraw the needle until **pulsating** arterial blood fills your syringe.
11. If you withdraw the needle almost to the skin surface without obtaining blood, don't pull the needle all the way out. Instead, palpate the artery again, redirect your needle, and thrust again. This saves the patient from another skin puncture.
12. Grab the gauze pad, remove the needle, and compress the puncture site tightly for at least four minutes. You can ask a reliable patient to compress the site. *If the site is not compressed, the patient will get a hematoma.*
13. Eliminate all air bubbles by inverting the syringe, tapping, and squirting.
14. Discard the needle safely.
15. Quickly cover the syringe with a stopper and put the specimen on ice.

> If arterial blood is not kept on ice, cells consume the oxygen and alter pH and pCO2, making results inaccurate.

16. Clean up.
17. Make sure the requisition include correct patient identity, temperature, and inspired oxygen concentration.

> "RA" means the patient is breathing room air; 2 liters N.C. means the patient's air is supplemented with 2 liters/min of oxygen via nasal cannula; 50% means the FiO2 is just that.

18. Deliver the specimen to the blood gas lab or have the "stat messenger" called. Make sure the specimen is actually picked up.

Electrocardiograms

Obtaining an ECG (aka EKG) is one of the most valuable things a JMS can do during an emergency like an impending cardiac arrest.

A standard twelve-lead ECG has five or ten electrodes which are color-coded. Memorize these codes. Green means right leg (the leg you use for the gas pedal on a car); red means left leg (the leg closest to the brake pedal); white means right arm (it rhymes); black means left arm. There are either one (labeled V) or six (labeled V1 - V6) electrodes for the chest leads, and they are all brown. Always apply the limb (non-brown) leads first, so a preliminary rhythm strip can be obtained quickly). *In case of amputation or cast, apply the electrode to the neareset shoulder or groin.*

Chest leads are applied as follows: V1 at the fourth right intercostal space adjacent to the sternum, V2 at the corresponding fourth left intercostal space, V4 at the fifth intercostal space along the midclavicular line, V3 exactly midway between V2 and V4 (**not** near the umbilicus), V5 at the fifth intercostal space along the anterior axillary line, V6 at the fifth intercostal space along the midaxillary line. If there is only one chest electrode, you need to move it and record each precordial lead individually. Adhesive electrode pads are easiest.

Good electrical contact is essential between electrodes and skin. You can't make good contact on hairy places, so find bald places on limbs. Occasionally you may need to shave or even abrade particularly hairy spots.

> **Be sure electrodes make good electrical contact with skin.**

Make sure the patient stays absolutely still while you are obtaining the actual ECG. Don't hold any electrodes in place, and don't touch the patient. Make sure the ECG machine is set for 1 mV/cm (sensitivity = 1) and 25mm/sec unless you specifically want something else.

Every Junior Medical Student should read Dale Dubin's nearly-out-of-print "Rapid Interpretation of EKGs" from Cover Publishing Company. It is simply the best introduction available, and it will get you up to speed in a few hours.

Always interpret the ECG as soon as it is obtained. Don't just look at the computer interpretation. Vital information should not languish in your pocket.

Lumbar Puncture

A discussion of how to perform lumbar puncture is beyond the scope of this guide. Once you obtain the cerebrospinal fluid, you may need assistance submitting the specimens to the laboratory. Generally, four or five tubes are collected, each containing 1-2mL, and numbered in the order they were collected.

Two separate tubes (usually the first and the last) are submitted to hematology for cell count. If the CSF contains blood from the trauma of LP, the later tube is expected to contain many fewer cells.

Another tube (usually the second) is submitted for culture. Ordinarily CSF is cultured only for bacteria, but if there is a clinical suspicion, it should be submitted for mycobacterial, viral, or fungal culture. Latex agglutination tests are available for rapid assay of cryptococcus and of encapsulated bacteria in CSF.

Another tube (usually the third) is submitted to the chemistry lab for protein and glucose determination.

Finally, you should always try to save a specimen of CSF in the refrigerator. That way if a specimen is lost, or if you decide you need additional tests (like protein electrophoresis or cryptococcal antigen), you won't need to repeat the LP

> Submitting CSF specimens
>
> Tubes 1 & 4: Cell count   Tube 3: Protein, glucose
>
> Tube 2: Culture, gram stain   Tube 5: Save in refrigerator

When you perform an LP, you should also perform laboratory tests on the CSF. You should do a cell count, and if indicated, a Gram stain looking for organisms and cells. You should also make an India ink preparation to look for cryptococcus.

> Add a drop of serum to CSF when preparing a gram stain.

"Bedside" gram stains of CSF can be problematic: if the CSF protein is low, the specimen probably will not adhere to the glass slide and you may miss cells and organisms. Try spinning down some blood and adding a drop of serum to the CSF specimen before staining.

Nasogastric Tube (NG) and Dobhoff placement

Indications
- Suction of gastric secretions in patients with bowel ileus or obstruction.
- Diagnostic lavage of gastric hemorrhage.
- Enteral alimentation.

Supplies

- Nasogastric suction tube (vented) or "Salem Sump."

    - or -

    Dobhoff-style weighted feeding tube with matching stylet. Insert the stylet all the way into the Dobhoff tube.

- Water-soluble lubricant (*e.g.*, Surgilube brand)
- 50mL syringe
- Glass of ice water and straw
- Chux
- Cloth tape
- Gloves

Placing an NG or Dobhoff tube

1. Estimate the distance a tube would have to travel between the patient's nostril and epigastrium. Note which marker on the tube corresponds to this distance.
2. Put a generous amount of lubricant on the proximal 5 or 10 cm of the tube.
3. Discuss what is about to happen with the patient. For example, say: "A lubricated tube will be passed into the nose and throat where it will tickle and perhaps hurt, then you will be asked to swallow water while the tube is inserted into the stomach. You may cough or gag temporarily, but your cooperation is important."
4. Ask the patient to sit upright, tilting the head forward.
5. Put on gloves. Place chux underneath the patient's face.
6. Inspect the nostrils with a pen light, avoiding the one toward which the septum deviates.
7. Insert the lubricated tube into the nostril, aiming posteriorly and slightly **inferiorly**, not the along the upward course of the nasal passage.

> Aim downwards in the nasopharynx.

8. Advance the tube until the patient gags or you encounter some resistance.
9. Ask the patient to start drinking water through the straw. Advance the tube further while the patient drinks. By swallowing, the patient closes the epiglottis and drives the tube into the esophagus. Continue advancing until you reach the distance you estimated earlier.
10. If the tube won't advance, make sure it isn't coiled in the posterior pharynx. Check inside the patient's mouth. Withdraw and try again.
11. If the patient continues to gag and choke incessantly, the tube may be in the trachea. Withdraw the tube and try again.

> Rule of thumb: a patient usually can't speak with an NG tube in the trachea.

12. Check to make sure the tube is in the stomach. Using the syringe, blow 50mL of air into the stomach while listening to the epigastrium with a stethoscope. You should hear the air bubbling through the stomach.
13. Secure the tube to the patient's nose using cloth tape. I like to rip a 2x1" strip of tape longitudinally for half it's length, placing the intact half on the tip of the nose, and wrapping each arm of the tape around the tube.
14. Do not remove the guidewire from a Dobhoff tube until you obtain the radiograph below. Also, never replace a guidewire into a Dobhoff once you have withdrawn it; the wire may slide out of the Dobhoff tube and may perforate a viscus.
15. Obtain a STAT portable KUB radiograph to make sure the distal end of the tube is in the stomach and not in a lung.

> Always check Dobhoff placement with a radiograph.

16. Once the KUB shows the tube in the correct location, remove the guidewire from the Dobhoff tube. Notify the nurses that the tube is ready for use.

Placing a Urinary (Foley) Catheter

It is important to remember that urinary catheterization, especially chronic, is associated with substantial morbidity. Bladder catheters violate the integrity of the urinary sphincter and provide a mode of entry for bacteria colonizing and infecting the urinary tract. The risk of urinary tract infection grows with the duration of bladder catheterization. There is also the risk of damaging the urinary outflow tract, superficially as in simple epithelial tears causing gross hematuria, or seriously, as in trauma patients with unrecognized urethral disruption.

There is no question that urinary catheters are convenient, both for patients and for nurses. But in light of the above risks, especially of infection, it is important to review the indication for every patient's ongoing urinary catheterization every day.

> Review the indication for ongoing Foley catheters every day. Remove the catheter if the risk of continued use outweighs the benefit.

Common indications for urinary catheters
Monitoring
- Hemodynamic monitoring in critically ill patients.
- Monitoring urine output in oliguric patients.
- Inability to void spontaneously.
- Urinary outflow obstruction (*e.g.,* severe prostatism), both for diagnosis and for therapy.

> Check postvoid residuals when outflow obstruction is suspected: The patient tries to empty the bladder completely. Then a urinary catheter is placed and the residual urinary volume is measured. More than 50-100mL suggests obstruction.

- Chronic urinary incontinence (*e.g.,* after spinal cord injury, severe neurogenic bladder).
- Temporary urine collection.
  - In severely debilitated patients unable to use a bedpan or toilet.
  - When otherwise unable to collect a sterile specimen for culture.
  - In extremely large-volume diuresis (to spare the patient from too-frequent voiding, *e.g.,* in cancer chemotherapy).

Protection
- Maintain patency of urethra after urologic procedures or when blood clots are passed from urinary tract.
- Protect surrounding perineum when urinary soilage would be detrimental *(e.g.,* with severe decubiti).
- Bladder lavage with medications (*e.g.,* amphotericin B).

Supplies for urinary catheterization
- Catheters:

  Straight catheters are intending for insertion, urine collection, and immediate removal.

  Foley or **indwelling** catheters are intended to be left in place for some period of time. They have an inflatable balloon near the tip to keep them from slipping out of the bladder. **Coudé-tip** Foley catheters have a special tapered/curved end to facilitate passage in men with enlarged prostates.

  Irrigation catheters are Foley catheters with an additional port for infusion of irrigation fluid, like amphotericin for candidal cystitis.

- Sterile gloves
- Povidone-iodine swabs and sterile towels to prepare a sterile field.
- Lubricant jelly.
- Water-filled syringe to inflate the Foley balloon, if needed.
- Foley catheter collection bag, if needed.

Placing the urinary catheter
Most people use the technique of keeping one gloved hand "sterile" to manipulate the catheters, and the other gloved hand "contaminated" to hold the genitals and prevent contamination of the Foley catheter.

1. Spread "chux" pads liberally on bed to minimize the mess.

> Keep one hand "sterile" and one hand "contaminated."

2. With your "contaminated hand," hold the glans penis or spread the labia majora to expose the urethra. You will keep your contaminated hand in this position throughout the procedure.
3. With your clean hand, prepare the urethral meatus and surrounding area with povidone-iodone.

4. Apply the sterile towel to prepare a sterile field.
5. With your "sterile" hand, insert the **lubricated** catheter into the urethra.
6. In men, hold the glans penis anterosuperiorly, as if it were erect.
7. Insert the catheter all the way until urine appears. Keep inserting the **catheter up to the hub**, to avoid balloon inflation while within a segment of the urethra.
8. In some patients, prostatic enlargement interferes with urethral catheterization. If you encounter urethral resistance, first try gentle pressure. If this fails, a special *Coudé*-tip catheter easily will pass the prostate in men.

> Always insert the Foley catheter entirely to the hub before inflating the balloon!

9. Apply the water-filled syringe to inflate the Foley balloon. Pay attention to the patient; if balloon inflation causes pain, something is wrong.
10. Apply gentle traction to the Foley catheter to bring the balloon against the bladder wall.
11. Connect the Foley catheter to the urine collection bag.
12. Clean up.

Procedure Notes

Every time a bedside procedure is performed, a procedure note should be left in the chart. Aside from the legal implications, this lets others know when specific lines were placed, when specific specimens were obtained, *etc.* Procedure notes are miniature operative notes, consisting of:

- Procedure performed. Date & time.
- Indications for the procedure.
- Documentation that the indications and risks were explained to the patient and that the patient consented.

- Relevant lab tests.
- Anesthesia used, if any.
- A brief description of the procedure.
- Complications and estimated blood loss.
- How patient tolerated the procedure.
- Specimen obtained.

> Example:
> 3/15/2020 23:15
> Procedure: Lumbar puncture.
> Indications: R/O meningitis.
> Informed consent was obtained.
> PT: 12.0 sec; Plt 175k.
> Sterile prep, 1% lidocaine local, lateral decubitus position. 22G spinal needle into L3-L4 subarachnoid space and 4mL of clear cerebrospinal fluid was obtained. Opening pressure 180 mm.
> EBL negligible.
> Patient tolerated procedure well.
> CSF sent for cell count, gram stain, bacterial and fungal culture, protein, and glucose.

Local Anesthesia

For many procedures, subcutaneous lidocaine is given for anesthesia. Anesthesia techniques are beyond the scope of this guide, but here are a few comments:

- It rarely makes sense to instill lidocaine for a procedure that otherwise requires a single needlestick, like IV placement.
- Lidocaine preparations are available that contain small amounts of epinephrine (2% lidocaine, 1:100,000 epinephrine). These usually are labeled in red. Epinephrine is an intense local vasoconstrictor and will reduce local bleeding. This can ease closure of a wound, for example. Do not use lidocaine with

epinephrine on extremities, where vasoconstriction may cause severe necrosis.

- Do not reuse multiple-use lidocaine vials. Do not use lidocaine with epinephrine on the face or extremities. Lidocaine preparations often come in multiple-use containers. The savings these vials offer are outweighed by the dangers: some physicians inadvertently use blood-contaminated needles to withdraw lidocaine from these vials. Do not risk transmitting blood-borne disease by re-using multiple-use vials.
- Always check if a patient is allergic to lidocaine before administering it.

Imaging Tests

Medical imaging, whether performed by diagnostic imaging services (aka radiology) or by point-of-care imaging services (such as obstetrics or cardiology), has become profoundly important and expensive. Not to mention unpleasant, time-consuming, and expensive for your patients.

Some of your greatest medical harms and worst medical errors will be directly related to medical imaging misadventures. Trust me.

Make a lifetime habit of directly reviewing every medical imaging examination you ever request on your patients. Do not rely on the intentionally ambiguous language of specialists. Do not wait until you develop your own imaging expertise. Start immediately. Trust me.

Bedside Tests

A note from the past about bedside tests...
Since this book was first written, the CLIA quality assurance law and occupational safety considerations have made it difficult for students and physicians to perform their own bedside tests.

This should not stop you from trudging to the laboratory to review actual blood urine sputum and related specimens using your own self, on every patient. It will make you a better doctor!

Urinalysis

Kidneys are our friends. The physical exam is limited but there is a wealth of information to be gleaned from direct inspection of urine.

Collecting Urine
You can't perform a good test without a good specimen. Urine should be freshly collected when you test it. After sitting around for more than a half-hour or so, cellular elements and casts decompose and bacteria may overgrow the specimen. So try to act quickly. Refrigerate urine to be submitted to the hospital laboratory.

> Urine specimens must be tested quickly after collection. Urine specimens not obtained cleanly or submitted fresh can be "overgrown" by bacteria not causing infection.

Ambulatory patients
Ask the patient to wipe the urethral meatus with povidone-iodine (Betadine) and then wipe dry with a clean cloth. Remind women to wipe from front to back. Have the patient initiate a urine stream without catching the initial urine and then catching about 30mL of midstream urine; this technique discards urethral- and genital-contaminated material. Instruct the patient how to handle to specimen container so as not to contaminate it.

Patients using bedpans
Help these patients wipe the urethral meatus as above and catch the midstream urine. Avoid collecting urine from the bedpan itself, if possible. You may need the help of a nurse.

Patients who need urinary catheterization
If a patient cannot cooperate or if they cannot produce urine given a reasonable period of time, it may be appropriate to catheterize the bladder in sterile fashion (see page 110).

Foley catheter bags are designed to collect urine over hours or days in a "closed system." When left at the bedside, Foley bags quickly get overgrown with bacteria, confounding your urinalysis. Here's how to collect fresh specimens. Foley catheters have a latex-covered side port near the urethra through which you can stick a needle and withdraw urine into a syringe. Make sure you wipe the latex port with alcohol so as not to contaminate the urine collection system. Then use a large-bore (18G or larger) needle and *slowly* withdraw the urine to minimize disruption of urinary sediment, especially casts.

Collect fresh urine specimens from the collection sideport of Foley catheters.

Prepare the specimen for testing
1. Submit 10 ml to the hospital laboratory for culture. Find out what tube to use at your institution.
2. Put a drop of un-spun urine onto a glass microscope slide and cover it with a coverslip.
3. Sample the urine with a dipstick, following the instructions on the dipstick box for timing of interpretation (See below). You can dip the urine you plan to examine manually, but obviously you shouldn't put a dipstick into the specimen you will submit for culture.
4. Pour 5-10 ml into a centrifuge tube. Balance the centrifuge (with a tube of water) and spin your specimen at the proper setting (usually 1500-2500 rpm) for 3-5 minutes. Try not to

over-centrifuge the specimen, since most clinical centrifuges get pretty hot and damage cellular material.

5. Carefully pour off the supernatant from the centrifuge tube. Some people advise "flicking" the pellet to resuspend this; in my experience this technique disrupts almost all cellular casts. Instead you should use a Pasteur pipette carefully to transfer some of the pellet onto two glass slides: one for wet-mount and another for Gram stain.

> Don't "flick-resuspend" the sediment pellet; transfer sediment to a slide using a Pasteur pipette.

Chemical urinalysis: dipsticks and such

Modern dipsticks are so fancy that unless renal disease is strongly suspected, microscopic urinalysis is not warranted in the absence of dipstick abnormality. Conversely, you **must** examine the urine under a microscope if the dipstick has any abnormality. Nevertheless, some dipstick abnormalities are of limited clinical significance except in specific instances.

> Perform manual microscopic urinalysis whenever the dipstick is abnormal.

- **pH:** Urinary pH varies substantially throughout a given day for any individual patient, so the test is usually not valuable. However, in the presence of systemic acidosis, a urinary pH less than 6.0 suggests impaired renal acidification, as in renal tubular acidosis. Unusually high pH values, greater than 9.0 often result from ammonia release by urea-splitting organisms.

- **Specific gravity:** This also varies considerably throughout the day. S.G. greater than 1.023 suggests normal urine concentrating ability. S.G. greater than 1.030 suggests relative dehydration. S.G. less than 1.010 in the presence of fluid restriction suggests impaired urinary concentrating ability.

> Dipsticks are insensitive for Bence-Jones protein and globulin. Use SSA.

- **Protein:** Numerous conditions cause proteinuria. You should be aware that urinary dipsticks are insensitive for non-albumin urinary proteins, like Bence-Jones proteins in multiple myeloma. Mixing urine with a solution of sulfosalicylic acid (SSA) will precipitate these other proteins.
- **Glucose:** Ascorbic acid usually inhibits this test for glycosuria. Dipsticks do not detect all common ketones.
- **Ketones:** Are found in patients not only with diabetic ketosis but also patients who are fasting or acutely ill. Note that dipstick reagents react only to acetone and acetoacetate, not to beta-hydroxybutyrate. Therefore a negative dipstick for ketones does not exclude ketonuria. Furthermore, ketones in the urine do not necessarily mean the patient has ketosis.
- **Blood:** Dipsticks detect both hemoglobin and myoglobin. Some dipsticks claim to distinguish the two, but I've never seen that work properly. You should rely on microscopic urinalysis to determine the presence or absence of RBC's.

> Wait one to five minutes after dipping in urine before interpreting the leukocyte esterase test.

- **Leukocyte esterase:** This enzyme test detects WBC's in urine, unreliably in my clinical experience. You should wait one to five minutes before reading the L.E. dipstick: that's considerably longer than the other dipstick reagents. Rifampin, nitrofurantoin, and Pyridium interfere with the assay.

> The combination of leukocyte esterase and nitrite yields a sensitive but nonspecific test for urinary tract infection, with good negative predictive value.

- **Nitrites:** Gram-negative organisms reduce urine compounds to nitrites; the assay helps identify patients with significant bacteriuria.

Microscopic Urinalysis

Examine urinary sediment at low- and high-power under the microscope. Since you usually look at unstained material, it often helps to move the microscope condenser away from your specimen slide, to increase contrast.

> Move the microscope condenser away from your slide to increase contrast.

Good urinalysis can be like an archaeological expedition. You can learn much about the patient's past, health and lifestyle from their urine.

Specific objects to look for in microscopic urinalysis

Squamous epithelial cells suggest genital contamination of the urine specimen. **Squamous epithelium**: When you see more than a few of these large cells with small central nuclei, your specimen is likely contaminated with genital contents, and bacteriuria may represent this contamination. Try to get another specimen.

Significant bacteriuria implies more than one organism per oil immersion field on unspun urine. **Bacteria**: Most urine specimens contain some bacteria, but for *significant* bacteriuria there usually must be enough organisms to reveal one per oil-immersion microscope field on *unspun* urine. If you suspect significant bacteriuria, look for white blood cells and then prepare a Gram stain of spun urine to help identify a predominant organism.

Five WBC's per hpf suggest pyuria in centrifuged urine. **White blood cells**: These have the typical multilobed nucleus. A few WBC's are not noteworthy, but more than 5 WBC's per high power microscope field suggest pyuria. It is said that neutropenic patients may have a urinary tract infection without significant pyuria. In the proper setting you may want to stain WBC's to look for eosinophils.

0-2 RBC's per hpf are normal in centrifuged urine. **Red blood cells**: Women (especially during menses) and catheterized patients are "allowed" to have a few (0-2) RBC's on their urinalysis. However if the abnormality persists on serial urinalyses they may need further evaluation for hematuria. Some observers attempt to distinguish RBC's from the bladder (which have normal morphology) from RBC's originating higher in the urinary tract (which may be *crenated* or distorted in the glomeruli or renal medulla).

Tubular epithelium: These cells are slightly larger than WBC's, and they appear elliptical with a small eccentric nucleus. An occasional tubular cell is not unusual but larger numbers suggest acute tubular necrosis. Clumps of tubular cells often degenerate into granular casts and debris; a mixture of these casts and tubular epithelial cells even better supports the diagnosis of acute tubular necrosis. Unfortunately, it may be difficult to distinguish tubular cells from transitional epithelial cells originating in the urinary collecting system, which have a similar appearance but are slightly larger and tapered.

Cellular casts are always abnormal and demand immediate attention. **Casts**: Cellular casts are always abnormal and suggest tubular or glomerular disease. The most common you see are *granular* casts, which are thought to represent "skeletons" of cells like WBC's, RBC's, and tubular cells. RBC casts suggest glomerulonephritis. WBC casts suggest pyelonephritis. Tubular casts suggest tubular injury. A few hyaline casts can be seen in normal people. Waxy casts may be normal in patients with chronic renal failure, but may also represent further degeneration of granular casts.

Crystals: A few oxalate crystals can be seen in normal (acid) urine; they are small squares with a refractile central cross. Larger numbers may reflect ethylene glycol ingestion, but the oxalate crystals in these patients often take the monohydrate form; they are slender spike-like and resemble uric acid crystals. Normal (alkaline) urine contains coffin-lid-shaped triple-phosphate crystals and calcium carbonate crystals. Other crystals are usually abnormal.

Other objects: flagellates, bacteria, fat, contaminants: You commonly see things like trichomonads, spermatozoa, and genital contaminants in urinalyses. Fat globules suggest fat embolization syndrome, not uncommon after orthopedic injury or surgery.

Gram Stain

Patients admitted to the hospital for infection need immediate diagnosis and therapy. Gram stains can help in diagnosing bacterial infection and in choosing the proper antibiotics empirically without waiting one to three days for cultures to definitively to identify causative organisms.

> You can significantly contribute to a patients care by speedily preparing a gram stain of infected material.

Preparing a specimen for Gram Stain

Use clean glass slides; dirt can cause confusion under the microscope. Wash the slide with alcohol or soap and water if necessary. Avoid excessive force when spreading material on the slide, which can disrupt or distort the cells you want to view. Here are some specific suggestions for different types of specimen:

Sputum: Place a small amount of sputum on a glass slide. Use a second glass slide to spread the material evenly and thinly. You end up with two slides, one good for Gram stain and the other for backup or for acid-fast bacillus staining. Let the slide air-dry before proceeding.

Urine: Use centrifuged sediment; gently spread it on a glass slide as above. Alternatively, place a drop of urine on the slide, permit it to dry, then place another drop over the first, repeating the cycle several times until a visible sediment is deposited. Air-dry.

Cerebrospinal fluid: Use the serial drop-then-dry method described for urine. As mentioned earlier, Gram stains of CSF can be problematic because when CSF protein is low, cells are easily washed off the slide during staining. One approach is to grab some serum by spinning down a blood specimen and adding a drop to the CSF to help it "stick" to the slide. Air-dry.

Pus: Prepare this just like you would sputum.

Before staining you must **heat-fix** the specimen to the slide. Pass the slide over a flame quickly, but make sure you don't "fry" your specimen by making the slide too hot. If it hurts when you touch it to the back of your hand, it's too hot.

Staining the Slide

In spite of what they may have taught you, it takes about as long to stain your specimen as it does to stain your finger: even a second will do the trick. So it should only take a few moments to prepare a good Gram stain. The most challenging part is proper decolorizing.

Find a sink and hold the slide while you pour reagents over it. Get it?

Gram Crystal violet: Flood the slide with crystal violet reagent. It's that simple.

Rinse: Use ordinary tap water. Be careful not to let the water stream wash your specimen off the slide. I like to let the stream fall on my gloved thumb and from there gently rinse the slide.

Gram Iodine: Again, just flood the slide. You don't need to wait before you again **rinse**.

Gram decolorizer: This stage is critical. Make sure you use 95% alcohol or an alcohol-acetone mix, not acid-alcohol designed for decolorizing acid-fast bacillus (AFB) stains.

Decolorize just until the iodine stops moving into the alcohol rinse. Watch this by holding the slide over a light background. Flood the slide with alcohol and hold it somewhere in the room so there is a light-colored background behind the slide. You should see excess iodine stain dissolving into the alcohol. Pour off the alcohol, rinse, and apply some more alcohol. You should continue this (usually 10-30 seconds) just until you stop seeing more iodine stain dissolving into the alcohol. *Rinse immediately.*

If you don't rinse properly, the slide will be under-decolorized or over-decolorized and therefore may be difficult to interpret. You will see that specimens spread on the slide too thickly or too unevenly are difficult to decolorize.

Safranin: This is a red counterstain designed to stain all of the other material on the slide. Again, just flood the slide and **rinse**.

Dry: Either blot the slide on blotting paper, let it dry in the warm-dry incubator nearby, or just be patient.

Interpreting the Gram Stain

Check for contamination. Under low-power look for squamous epithelial cells. If you find them, especially with sputum, the specimen is probably contaminated with normal flora; oral and throat organisms in sputum, genital organisms in urine. You should probably discard the specimen and start again. Culture results also will probably not be helpful in this setting.

Find the area of interest. Under low power, find an area laden with inflammatory cells.

Switch to an oil-immersion lens. Properly stained slides have PMN's with pinkish, not purple or pale, nuclei.

Determine adequacy of staining. Properly Gram-stained specimens show WBC's with pink-red nuclei. If the nuclei are pale, the specimen is probably over-decolorized and Gram positive organisms may appear Gram-negative. If the nuclei are purplish-blue (more common), the specimen is probably under-decolorized, and Gram negative organisms may appear Gram positive. Note that you can take any slide and further decolorize it with alcohol; just repeat the safranin counterstain stage.

Look for them around clusters of WBC's, or even inside WBC's.

> **Identify Gram-negative and Gram-positive organisms.** Once you find Gram-positive organisms, take special care to look further for Gram-negative ones.

Purple organisms are Gram-positive; pink organisms are Gram-negative. You should know that finding Gram-positive organisms is psychologically distracting; you may stop looking at the slide systematically and you may actually miss sheets of Gram-negative organisms.

Determine the morphology. Decide if the bacteria are *bacilli* (rods) or *cocci* (spherical). See whether *cocci* are in pairs (*diplococci*), chains (*streptococci*), or clusters (*staphylococci*). Some people like to divide gram-negative *bacilli* morphologically into those which are plump (possibly enteric), those which are filamentous (possibly *hemophilus* or *pseudomonas*), and those which are pleiomorphic (having varying shapes, as with *hemophilus*).

Some organisms have classic shapes and can be identified with some accuracy just from the Gram stain. *Pneumococci* typically are lancet-shaped Gram-positive *diplococci*, with colinear long-axes. *Neisseria*, including *gonococcus* and *meningococcus* are similar-appearing Gram-negative diplococci, except the long-axes are parallel instead of colinear. Gram-positive cocci in clusters are usually *staphylococcus* species. Gram-negative pleiomorphic rods, especially in sputum or CSF, are often *hemophilus* species. Gram-positive rods in foul-smelling pus suggest *clostridia* species. The absence of organisms in the presence of WBC's on Gram stain can be helpful also. For instance, in a patient with clinical pneumonia, purulent sputum, and WBC's without visible organisms may suggest an "atypical pneumonia" caused by *legionella* or *mycoplasma* organisms.

Organize

Organizing your data and your schedule

You need to keep track of a vast array of changing information about your patients. Good organization is essential. Below are a few popular ways in which students and house officers keep track of patient data. Mix and match to suit your taste.

Protect confidentiality

Your documents, whether paper or electronic, are confidential unofficial medical records. Laws, including HIPAA, apply. Treat them, and dispose of them, with care.

Index Cards or Electronic Equivalent

Three-by-five index cards, or applications such as EverNote are handy because you can keep all the patient info you need in your pocket. You can unobtrusively palm your note cards or device while you present your patients to your team and your attendings. And you can keep your old cards for future reference or in case your patients get readmitted to the hospital.

Stamp your note cards with the patient name and ID number at the ward desk. Most people can fit a good summary of the H&P on a single 3x5 index card. Make sure to include the admission problem list.

Some people put patient info on the front of the card, and put lab data all on the back of the card. Others keep taping additional cards, with more detailed information, to the back of the "master" index card.

If you don't like to write and read microscopically, you can keep a separate sheet on your clipboard with all the information others keep on a 3x5 card. Just a matter of style.

Master sheets

As you may have noticed, time available for patient care is very limited. It is very important therefore to keep track of all of the tasks that need to be performed each day.

Some people like to keep daily checklists of tasks on each individual patient card or sheet. I don't like this technique, because in a busy hospital it is difficult to accomplish all tasks on patients one at a time. Instead I much prefer keeping a daily "master sheet" of all tasks to be accomplished and new information acquired. This way I can tell "at a glance" what remains to be done, and I take advantage of "idle" time.

Paper can be much better than personal electronic devices, because of the ability to depict the "big picture." I use a two-dimensional grid. Along the vertical axis I write the names of all of my patients, with the sickest and most recently-admitted near the top. I keep the following headings along the horizontal axis:

Problem list. The exhaustive admission diagnostic evaluation generates a list of problems. Your goal-oriented daily plan should address every active problem. Follow this list carefully whenever you talk about the patient on rounds.

Physical findings. Record new physical findings, morning vital signs, 24° maximum temperature, weight, and fluid balance. Circle the findings you need to review with your supervisors.

To-do list. Leave the most room here. It includes everything you have to do before going home. Usually your resident adds to this list every morning on work rounds. For example, call social worker to arrange family meeting to discuss placement, perform corticotropin stimulation test, replace IV, call cardiology consult, *etc.* Cross off tasks as you accomplish them.

Labs and new data. Every time you order a new lab test, leave blank space in this area. In your idle time, when you see the blankness on your sheet you can check the computer or lab to see if the results are available. When you get the results, record them here proudly. Do the same thing for other tests, like radiological studies and new advice from consultants.

- **Reading topics.** Reading about the problems your patients face is the best way to learn about medicine. Ordinarily dull topics become suddenly interesting, you are far more likely to remember what you read, and you are better prepared to take care of the patients. Dozens of issues come up every day on every patient. Try to keep a list of these topics on your master sheet. At the end of the day try to look up a reasonable fraction of these topics.

This technique can make anyone into a compulsive, truly excellent Junior Medical Student. Once you fill-in-the-blanks of this daily master sheet, it is a breeze to write your daily progress note. All of your data is on-hand, along with every topic you need to address in your note. Similarly, your sheet is a great cue-card for organizing your presentations on morning work rounds. Your team will appreciate your organized and smooth presentations, and they will give you more attention and responsibility when they see you doing such a good job.

At the end of every day, **re-write** a fresh master sheet for the next day, with problem lists and leftover "to-do's." Your morning will be far more organized this way. You may also want to copy your daily lab data onto your index cards.

Presentations

As a Junior Medical Student you face a double standard for oral presentations. You are expected to be thorough yet nearly as brief as every other time-conscious member of the team. Even if you don't have an enchanting personality, you can make truly excellent presentations if you follow a few precepts:

> Have all data on-hand. Confirm all observations and reports yourself.

Know everything about your patient. Do not rely on others to supply data. It is bad form to ask your intern, in the middle of a presentation, what the electrocardiogram shows. Supply firsthand interpretations of tests, not just others' interpretations. Don't recite the official radiology report; instead describe what you found on the radiograph. And remember to include vital signs, always.

Structure presentations around your problem list or differential diagnosis. A good presentation leads your listeners to your conclusions effortlessly. This takes considerable advance planning.

Avoid extraneous information. People stop listening when you talk about normal tonsils in a patient admitted for uremia; once that happens, they may be distracted from your important observation of Ewart's sign.

Memorize as much as you can. Your presentations will be much smoother when you have to rely on notes only for cues and not for words. You won't only appear to have a greater grasp of your patients' care; you will.

Don't waffle about your observations. Don't say, "I think she maybe had a question of jugular venous distention." Either she has JVD or not; either you recognized it or you didn't. If you are not sure, say simply "I think she has JVD," and review the finding at the bedside.

Don't use jargon, unless you are completely comfortable with the terminology. Invariably a JMS sounds awkward using technical terms inappropriately when simple English would suffice.

It should not surprise you that your admission note or progress note, carefully abbreviated, will serve as a good script for oral presentations.

For each patient you follow, you should be prepared to make several kinds of oral presentations. You will need to present new patients differently to house staff and to attendings. You will also need to report daily progress on rounds.

Presenting New Patients to House Staff

New patients admitted to the service are presented to the rest of the house staff team, usually during morning work rounds. You need to communicate every important item in less than three minutes. If you take longer, your team will grow impatient, and your resident may cut you off. If you are sloppy, your intern may need to interrupt you and supply details. Prepare notes or practice your presentations in advance, if you need to. Try to include the following, not necessarily in the same format:

- The patient's name, age, and sex. You may prefer to include relevant items of the past medical history in the same breath. For example, "He is a 74 year old man with long-standing hypertension and *diabetes mellitus* here because of a single syncopal episode on the morning of admission."

- Why the patient sought medical attention, and the duration of symptoms. You need to state this carefully in order to plant

the seed of your (already assembled) differential diagnosis in your listeners.
- Highlights of the history of present illness.
- Relevant details of the past medical history.

Remember: Pertinent positives and pertinent negatives.

- Medications and allergies.
- Skip the review of systems. Review positives with your resident afterwards.
- Restrict social and family history to essentials.
- Physical exam including appearance, vital signs, and positive physical findings. Most residents are grateful when you say "the head and neck exam was normal" if in fact it was.

If you don't quickly supply an impression and plan, your resident may assume you don't have one.

- Pertinent laboratory results. Ask your resident how much you should supply.
- Your problem list.
- Your brief impression and differential diagnosis.
- Your brief diagnostic and therapeutic plans.

Remember that you must provide all of the above information in about three minutes.

Presenting New Patients to Attendings
These presentations are very similar to the ones you make to housestaff, only longer. Usually these presentations take ten to fifteen minutes. Don't worry, you still will face the problem of choosing material to omit. Ask your attending how complete you should be, or how much time you have.

Most importantly, you should leave enough time to provide a detailed problem list, differential diagnosis, and assessment, particularly on internal medicine. You will learn more if you explain your thought processes, and your attending-led discussions will be livelier.

Looking Good
Here are a few personal suggestions on how to do an especially good job as a medical student.

Know your patients
This is the single most important piece of advice. You have more time to gather information about your patients than do interns and residents. You should know everything about them, past and future. And you should be responsible for every management chore on the patients you follow. That means:

Beat the intern to all tasks. If blood needs to be drawn, you should draw it. If lines need to be placed, you should place them. If a medication needs to be ordered, you should write the order. Interns have a hurried schedule; if you don't act fast, they will hustle things along on their patients without you. Conversely, house officers will love you for lightening their workload by getting jobs done without them.

Learn about test results as soon as they are available. If your patient gets a CT scan, go down to radiology, look at the film, and ask a radiologist for help interpreting it. If a crucial lab test has been sent, find out when the results will be returned and report them as soon as they are available. This way you will be "in the thick of things" and you will be better able to participate in management. As I mentioned elsewhere, it is uncool to ask an intern "what did the ECG show?" in the middle of a presentation.

Spend time with your patients. See them several times a day. Get to know them and their concerns. Examine them thoroughly every time you see them. Repeat history-taking with them every day until every element of their history is clear.

Work Hard during Night Call
There are two schools of thought about working hard on call as a student. One maintains that if you stay up late, you may be too tired

to concentrate effectively the next day, to study, and to impress attendings. The other school (which happens to be mine) says, if you stay up late, you will learn much more, you will gain more confidence, and you probably will earn more responsibility and attention. Here are a few tidbits.

- **Pick up new patients early.** That way you can complete your workup and note early in the evening and concentrate on all of the other ward activities.

- **Don't be too picky about patients.** As a student you have much to learn from every single patient who gets admitted to the hospital, even if it is your fifth patient with congestive heart failure.

- **Perform (or at least view) all bedside tests on all patients you admit.** On every patient you admit to a medical or pediatric service, you should personally do urinalyses, Gram stains, and peripheral smears. Most of these tests are difficult to interpret without direct experience. This is the best opportunity you will have to get experience. Note that many house officers do not do some of these tests themselves, but rely on laboratory interpretations or misinterpretations. If you are really good, you should do all bedside tests on all patients admitted to your service at night. Your intern will love you, and you will become very competent.

Consider not writing the admission note immediately. This may be hard, but you may miss much excitement if you scurry off to write your note. You may do well to wait until later in the evening, when things settle down on the wards.

Rule of thumb: interns who "scut you to death" tend to be bad doctors and bad teachers. Stay away!

Try to assume responsibility for a certain amount of "scut" tasks. I think few tasks are not educational for students. You might offer to do a fraction of the blood cultures and IV's that need to be done. The experience can be valuable. Interns will appreciate the extra effort you make to help them and they will make an effort to help you.

Speed your patients' care. If your patient needs a CT/LP, don't let them wait an hour for the requisition to be delivered and for the transporter to arrive. Take the req and the patient down to radiology, watch the CT, participate in its interpretation, and bring the patient back to the floor for the LP. This can save hours, and your patients will have gotten better care. By the same token, run specimens to the laboratory personally to make sure important jobs get done.

"Tag along" with your intern after your floor work is done. See how the intern admits patients and does procedures. Watch how the intern approaches acute problems on "cross-coverage" patients, whom the intern does not know well. Imagine yourself facing the same decisions as your intern. You will learn a lot.

What house officers like in a JMS
Think about it! What kind of student would you want around you if you were a harried intern? Would you like someone fumbling over him or herself to make a good impression? Or someone who can just let it hang loose? Would you want a student who seems bored by what you do, or inattentive when you try to explain things, or unavailable when help is needed, or busy writing notes when exciting things are happening with patients? Housestaff tend to like these qualities:

- Good & sympathetic company.
- Enthusiasm for every task.
- Students who lighten the workload, not add to it.
- Students who help organize tasks, like keeping follow-up lists, checking lab data, *etc.*
- Students who gather important clues from patients that were missed by house officers.

What house officers don't like in a JMS
Having to ask a student to do something more than once.

Disorganized or lengthy presentations.

Students who complicate patient management by supplying inappropriate information (*e.g.,* "You probably won't survive the week") to the patient or unreliable information to the team.

Students who take better care of notes than of patients.

Students who attend lectures more compulsively than they care for patients.

Students who ask interns to delay tasks (*e.g.,* writing orders, doing procedures) but never stay around long enough to watch or help.

Self-righteous or pretentious students.

Students who are asleep on call nights. An exception is made for students who have any of the above faults.

Get off my lawn, kid!
Some cantankerous advice about jargon.

Most medical jargon is both pretentious and embarrassing. Even when used by senior medical staff. Imagine you are being observed by an anthropologist. Here are some common phrases that really get my bowels moving:

> A truly excellent JMS uses the national language, not jargon.

"The patient is a poor *historian*." You are the historian.

"This is a 35 year-old *female*." Of what species? Don't distance yourself from the little people. You are trying to become a physician. The patient is a 35 year-old woman.

"He *denies* chest discomfort." Why are you accusing him? If the patient says he has no chest discomfort, that is what you report. If you suspect he is not being straightforward, raise your suspicion.

> Stop accusing your patients.

"I could not *appreciate* a diastolic murmur." Your gratitude is unwelcome. Can you hear the murmur or not?

"She *presented* with shortness of breath." Did she give a slide presentation? Does her presentation make you feel special? Surely you mean "she sought attention for shortness of breath."

"He *refused* valve replacement surgery." This implies recalcitrance. In fact he *declined* surgery perhaps because he is making the best personal choice.

"*NCAT* or *normocephalic and atraumatic*." I'm your patient has no stigmata of vaginal delivery 82 years ago upon his birth.

"He was *worked up* for pulmonary thromboembolism before he came here, so there must be some other explanation." Just because another physician considered an alternative diagnosis at another timepoint based on earlier clinical data does not absolve you of the obligation to revisit that consideration now. Diseases evolve. "Workups," especially by other physicians, often are premature or incomplete.

"She *ruled out* for myocardial infarction." Don't just declare what *isn't* wrong with the patient. Make a diagnosis. This patient may have had no evidence for myocardial infarction, but perhaps infarcted only two hours later because of "un-appreciated" preinfarction angina.

Good Luck!

I hope you will find this guide useful in getting started. Don't worry about making a good impression; worry about being thorough and about taking good care of your patients. All of the other good things will fall into place.

Index

A

Allen test, 103
Allergy, 25
Apgar score, 70, 72
Arterial blood gas, 89, 102, 103
Attending physician, 3, 10, 16, 51, 56, 136

B

Bacteriuria, 123
Blood culture, 100, 101, 102
Blood tubes, 90
Body substance isolation, 84

C

Casts, urinary, 124
Cerebrospinal fluid, 126, 129
Condition, 25
consultants, 131
Consultants, 10, 16, 20
Cranial nerves, 77
Crystals, urinary, 124
CSF. See Cerebrospinal fluid

D

Developmental history, 51
Developmental milestones, 74
Dextrose, 31, 33
Diagnosis, 24
Diet, 28, 29, 68
Dietitians, 6
Differential diagnosis, 49, 54, 133, 135, 136
Dipsticks, 121
Discharge summary, 19, 59
Dobhoff tube, 109

E

Electrocardiogram (ECG), 106
Emergency Department, 12, 36

F

Fellows, 10
Foley catheter. See Urinary catheter

G

Glasgow Coma Scale, 76
Gram stain, 126

H

HepLock, 96
Heplock flush, 97
History of present illness, 50
Hospital admission, 11
Hospitals Community, 2
  Teaching, 2, 10
  VA, 4
House officers, 3, 5
HPI, 50

I

Internal Medicine, 56
Interns, 2, 3, 8, 18
IV catheter, 30, 31, 96, 97, 98
IV fluids, 30, 31, 32, 33, 87
  Maintenance, 33

J

Jargon, 140

K

Ketones, 122

L

Laboratory tests, 20, 53
Laxatives, 46
Leukocyte esterase, 122
Lidocaine, 116
Local anesthesia, 116
Lumbar puncture, 107

M

Medical Students, 10
MTR, 23, 25, 43, 57

N

Needles, 88
  Butterfly, 89
Neurology, 76
Neurology examination, 76
NG tube, 108
Night call, 13, 137
Nitrites, 123
Note
  Admission, 14, 19, 49, 134, 138
  C-Section, 72
  Delivery, 70
  Discharge, 59
  Labor, 69
  Operative, 63
  Post-operative, 66
  Post-Partum, 72
  Pre-operative, 62
  Procedure, 115
  Progress, 20, 34, 38, 56, 57, 64, 80, 132, 134
Nurse practitioners, 8
Nurses, 1, 5, 27, 35
Nursing units, 4

O

Obstetrics, 69
Occupational therapists, 7
Orders, 22
  Activity, 27
  Admission, 24
  Discharge, 35
  Medication, 39
  Stat, 37

P

Pediatrics, 43, 73
Pharmacists, 7
Phlebotomy, 86, 87
Physical Exam, 51
Physician assistants, 8
Potassium, 32
Prescriptions, 38, 43
Presentations
  Oral, 19, 133, 134
PRN medications, 37, 42, 43
Problem list, 131
Procedures, 83
Psychiatry, 80

R

Radiology, 17, 20, 133
Reflex examination, 78
Residents, 1, 2, 9, 61
Respiratory rate, 27
Respiratory therapists, 6
Review of systems, 51
Rounds
  Attending, 16
  Pre-, 15
  Work, 15

S

Saline, 32
Sensory examination, 78
Sign-out, 17
SOAP format, 56
Social history, 51
Social workers, 7
Specific gravity, 121
Sputum, 126
Stat, 37, 106
Surgery, 61

T

Tourniquet, 86, 93

U

Urinalysis, 119, 120, 123
Urinary catheter, 28, 112, 114

V

Vaccinations, 73
Vacutainers, 89
Venipuncture, 91
Vital signs, 26, 52
Volume resuscitation, 32

W

Ward secretary, 5

Printed in Great Britain
by Amazon